The Ethics of Hospital Trustees

Hastings Center Studies in Ethics

A SERIES EDITED BY

Gregory Kaebnick and Daniel Callahan

This series of books, published by The Hastings Center and Georgetown University Press, examines ethical issues in medicine and the life sciences. Established in 1969, The Hastings Center, located in Garrison, New York, is an independent, nonprofit, and nonpartisan research organization. The work of the Center is mainly carried out through research projects, the publication of the *Hastings Center Report* and *IRB: A Review of Human Subjects Research*, and numerous workshops, conferences, lectures, and consultations. The Hastings Center Studies in Ethics series brings the ongoing research of The Hastings Center to a wider audience.

THE ETHICS
of
HOSPITAL
TRUSTEES

Bruce Jennings, Bradford H. Gray, Virginia A. Sharpe,
and Alan R. Fleischman

Editors

GEORGETOWN UNIVERSITY PRESS / Washington, D.C.

Georgetown University Press, Washington, D.C.
© 2004 by Georgetown University Press. All rights reserved.
Printed in the United States of America

10 9 8 7 6 5 4 3 2 1   2004

This book is printed on acid-free recycled paper meeting
the requirements of the American National Standard
for Permanence in Paper for Printed Library Materials.

Library of Congress Cataloging-in-Publication Data

The ethics of hospital trustees / Bruce Jennings, Bradford H. Gray, Virginia A. Sharpe,
and Alan R. Fleischman, editors.
    p.   cm. — (Hastings Center studies in ethics)
    ISBN 1-58901-015-9 (cloth : alk. paper)
    1. Hospital trustees—Professional ethics.   2. Hospital
trustees—United States.   I. Jennings, Bruce, 1949–   II. Series.
RA971.E89 2004
174.2–dc22   2003019806

CONTENTS

PART III
Trusteeship in Practice: Decisions and Systems

ACKNOWLEDGMENTS

THE EDITORS of this volume thank first the members of the hospital trustee ethics task force whose deliberations and commitment to the issues made this book possible. In particular, we are indebted to Dr. William Hubbard for his steady hand as chair of the task force and for his invaluable advice and support. We also wish to acknowledge gratefully the support and encouragement provided by William Stubing and the Greenwall Foundation. Strachan Donnelley of The Hastings Center had the original idea for a collaboration between Hastings and the New York Academy of Medicine, and Dr. Jeremiah Barondess, president of the Academy, has been very supportive of the project as well.

We are of course most grateful to the contributing authors of this volume. We thank them for their patience during the protracted process of completing the manuscript, and their excellent work speaks for itself in these pages.

Many colleagues on the staffs of our respective institutions provided help in the preparation of this book. We thank Heather Thompson, Michael Khair, Ellen McAvoy, and Denise Wong of The Hastings Center, and Linda Weiss of the New York Academy of Medicine.

INTRODUCTION

A Framework for the Ethics of Trusteeship

Bruce Jennings, Bradford H. Gray, Virginia A. Sharpe,
and Alan R. Fleischman

Access to care, the quality of care, patients' rights, and social justice are values affected today by the economic and organizational forces that shape and reshape health care systems and institutions. Although the ethical issues pertaining to managed care organizations have been widely discussed,[1] comparatively little attention has been paid in bioethics to the nature of the modern hospital as an institution; and neither bioethics nor scholarship on hospital governance has paid much attention to the ethical roles and responsibilities of those who are ultimately in charge of its governance—hospital trustees. As the institution and mission of the hospital change, so does its relationship with its principal stakeholders—patients and families, physicians, nurses, and other professional staff, nonprofessional staff, partnering or affiliated health care organizations, and finally the surrounding community the hospital serves.

As the relationships among these stakeholders change, the ethical challenges of hospital governance, policymaking, and trusteeship also change and become more subtle and difficult. Traditional legal frameworks and paradigmatic understandings of the role of the trustee[2] are no longer sufficient as guides to ethically responsible accountability and conduct. Recent examples of conflicts of interest and of hospitals that were poorly served by insufficiently informed and inattentive boards underscore the significance of the contemporary trustee's role. Decisions about closing or merging an institution—or even the sale to a for-profit purchaser—raise issues about where trustees' ethical responsibilities lie and how they should weigh the competing interests that are at stake.

In 1997, The Hastings Center and the New York Academy of Medicine began a two-year project on the Ethical Responsibilities of Not-for-Profit Hospital Trustees. The project was supported by the Greenwall Foundation of New York City.

Our research was built around two main activities: We conducted a series of lengthy in-person interviews with ninety-eight trustees and chief executive officers from fifteen not-for-profit hospitals of different sizes and types located in the greater New York metropolitan area. We also convened a project Task Force chaired by William Hubbard, former dean of the University of Michigan School of Medicine, and comprised of hospital trustees, executives, physicians, philosophers, social scientists, and representatives of leading professional associations representing hospitals and hospital leadership.

The Task Force met six times to discuss and debate the current state of hospital governance, the pressures not-for-profit hospital trustees face, and the hard choices they must often make. The Task Force also considered the values, cultural expectations, and historical traditions that inform the trustee role as background for developing a typology of ethical issues in hospital trusteeship and a set of principles and norms to address them.

The present volume grows out of the work of this project. The papers included here are both conceptual/philosophical and empirical/sociological in nature. The Hospital Trustee Ethics Project developed a set of principles grounded in the ethical relationships between the trustees and the hospitals' various stakeholders; these principles are presented in a separate paper, "Ethics and Trusteeship for Health Care: Hospital Board Service in Turbulent Times," and are summarized below.[3] In other chapters in this volume, various members of our research group and other scholars who were invited to submit commissioned papers examine these principles and their contexts of practical application in depth.

Our goal throughout the book is to show that the decisions made by hospital trustees and the actions of hospital boards do raise important ethical issues and that the ethical dimensions of trustee service should be more explicitly recognized and discussed. We hope to provoke and to contribute to such a discussion and to facilitate an ongoing interest in the topic of trustee ethics, both within the trustee community and in the broader discussion of medicine and health care in our society today. We aim in particular to clarify ethical concepts and principles pertinent to the activities of both individual trustees and boards.[4]

These concepts and principles do not arise in a historical or cultural vacuum; the "practice" of trusteeship has a history and a tradition. It has a social meaning and normative rules. It is something that can be done well or badly, responsibly or irresponsibly, beneficially or harmfully, conscientiously or carelessly. Being a hospital trustee is a voluntary service with heavy demands, and persons who give of their time and talents in this service should be esteemed. But it is a service that should never be undertaken lightly or in a pro forma manner. Organizations, including hospitals, sometimes find it difficult to recruit qualified candidates to serve on their boards. But the importance and responsibilities of this role should never be underestimated.

A Framework for the Ethics of Trusteeship

It is important to all of us that not-for-profit hospitals be governed well and trustees do their job well. Hospitals deal with the most fundamental matters of human well-being; their services are not just another commodity in the marketplace. By providing health care services of high quality, a hospital is an important community resource. Those who run not-for-profit organizations owe a fiduciary duty to the founders, benefactors, and donors who support the institution with an expectation that their money will be used in certain ways and for certain purposes. Not-for-profit hospitals also enjoy tax-exempt status in return for fulfilling certain public purposes, and thus those who govern these institutions have a responsibility to all citizens and taxpayers to ensure that these public purposes are realized. There is much with which trustees have been entrusted. These public and private fiduciary promises, implicit in each trustee's acceptance of appointment to the board, lay the foundation for a set of more specific ethical and legal duties incumbent on not-for-profit hospital trustees.

In a legal sense, not-for-profit trustees are not as highly regulated or as accountable as the directors of for-profit corporations, who are formally accountable to the shareholders who elect them. State attorneys general oversee the conduct of not-for-profit trustees, and they rarely use their regulatory power to interfere with board actions, except in cases of the most blatant misconduct and abuse of trust.[5] The law trusts trustees and provides a set of general guidelines for conscientious service. The legal obligations of hospital trustees can be summarized as a duty of care, a duty of obedience, and a duty of loyalty (cf. chapter 2 of this volume). The trustee must attend meetings and become informed enough to make reasonable, prudent decisions. A trustee must adhere to the mission of the hospital. A trustee must pursue the best interest of the hospital and not misuse his or her position to advance personal interests. The trustee must avoid conflicts of interest, engage in open decision making, and act with an independent mind and in a fiduciary spirit.

This emphasis in the law of trusts and trusteeship on personal, conscientious goodwill and ethical motivation comports well with the perspective of ethics. Together, legal and ethical traditions provide guidance and high expectations for trustees. Trustees must face many dilemmas and hard decisions in the governance of a hospital. Yet they do not face those tough choices without a tradition of values and purposes to guide them. The ethical heritage of hospital trusteeship is an anchor in troubled waters.

To focus on trustees as individuals is to identify only one side of the subject of trustee ethics. The most important decisions that trustees make are not made alone, but collectively, by boards of trustees acting in a corporate capacity. Trustee ethics therefore requires attention both to individuals who occupy the role and discharge the responsibilities of that role and to the way these individuals operate collectively as governing boards. If properly organized and functioning, a board can enable trustees together to accomplish things that no one trustee acting alone could hope to accomplish, and that no mere collection of individuals, if they were not properly organized, could accomplish.

It follows that paying attention to how boards are organized and function, and how trustees make collective decisions, is of the utmost importance. If hospital governance is to fulfill high standards of ethical conduct and to honor the trust that has been placed in it, then it is not enough to appeal to the ethical standards and conscience of individual trustees alone. For even conscientious individuals may find it difficult or impossible to perform well in an unsupportive environment. It is also necessary to examine how boards should function so that individual trustees can be and do what they should.

Although trusteeship is not strictly speaking a profession—indeed, it is one of the most significant bastions of civic volunteerism and amateurism remaining in our highly specialized society—the ethics of the hospital trustee has an affinity in many important ways with the ethics of professionals' roles. A "role" is a set of norms, social expectations, and values as well as a set of particular skills, functions, and competencies.

In the past, trustee ethics have been largely tacit. But these tacit understandings are being unraveled by the current health care marketplace and can no longer be taken for granted. Insofar as this trend cannot be simply reversed, it is all the more necessary to reestablish and revivify a sense of ethical mission and obligation for hospital trustees on an explicit ethical footing.

The roles and occupations that exist in a society can each be looked at from two complementary points of view. They can be considered both in terms of the social functions they perform and in terms of the ethical or cultural norms and values they embody. The ethics of trusteeship is a framework of normative expectations that constitute the role of trustee, much as physician ethics sets forth in a systematic way the normative expectations that society invests in its doctors, or as professional legal ethics contains the norms that society holds for its lawyers.

Like the professions, trustees are expected to adhere to ethical standards over and above what is called for by ordinary morality, and in return they are granted significant power and prerogatives. The problem is to organize the normative expectations and demands placed on trustees into a coherent and systematic framework.[6] We offer below one such framework, organized around four general principles.

PRINCIPLES OF ETHICAL TRUSTEESHIP

The four principles of ethical trusteeship are (1) fidelity to mission, (2) service to patients, (3) service to the community, and (4) institutional stewardship.

Fidelity to mission. The primary principle of the ethics of trusteeship can be stated as follows: *Trustees should use their authority and best efforts justly to promote the mission of the not-for-profit organization, and to keep that mission alive by interpreting its meaning over time in light of changing circumstances.* We call this the principle of fidelity to mission.

The mission of the organization governed by trustees is central to the ethics of the trustee role because it is the cornerstone of all the trustee's other responsibilities. The board exists to direct the organization, but the organization exists to pursue and fulfill a mission, a moral and social objective. Without the mission, there would be no trustee role in the first place.

It is important to interpret this principle broadly. Fidelity to mission should not be interpreted to mean that the exclusive role of the trustee is to perpetuate the past or to resist change. The "mission" is not necessarily the document that the organization refers to as its "mission statement." The true mission of an institution is rooted in the past and in the tradition of the institution, but it also points toward the future. A mission is a dynamic thing, an overriding purpose that changes with changing environment and circumstances, and trustees are faithful to it when they adopt an open-minded orientation. A mission does not interpret itself any more than it implements itself. It is in need of ongoing interpretation and reflection, much as is the Declaration of Independence in American political theory or the Constitution in American law.

Fidelity to mission must also be understood so that it is compatible with the demands of ordinary morality. Even a narrow mission would not give a trustee carte blanche to ignore either the law or the requirements of general morality. If one were a trustee of an organization whose traditional mission was written in terms that once implied racial or religious discrimination, then in light of today's moral norms and laws, the mission should be reinterpreted in such a way that such discrimination was neither implied nor tolerated. Hospitals in the United States, like virtually all other institutions, used to be racially segregated; trustees apparently once thought that their duty to the hospital's patients (at least its white patients) required segregated wards. But today, fidelity to mission is perfectly compatible with—indeed would be seen as requiring—racially integrated patient care settings.

When we apply this principle to the setting of the not-for-profit hospital, three aspects of mission come to the fore and suggest more specific principles of trustee ethics. The generic mission of the not-for-profit hospital is comprised of three objectives: to promote the health and well-being of patients, to be a civic and health resource for the community, and to be a place of respectful, well-managed, and competent health care provision. Thus in addition to the principle of fidelity to mission, trustee ethics in the hospital includes three principles of service: service to patients by providing medical, nursing, and allied health care; service to community by, among other things, promoting health; and service to the hospital through stewardship on behalf of that uniquely valuable social institution.

Service to patients. Fidelity to the hospital mission calls for trustees to adhere to a principle of service to patients and to their health needs: *Trustees should ensure that high-quality health care is provided to patients in an effective and ethically appropriate manner.*

This principle is a requirement of diligent oversight of management and of the hospital's performance. It also calls upon trustees to support the promotion of health in manifold ways, including by mobilizing resources for professional medical, nursing, and allied health services, by participating in professional education and biomedical research, by providing chronic and palliative care, and by sustaining a meaningful and dignified quality of life for patients.

It requires that trustees protect and promote the rights and interests of patients by maintaining hospital policies and procedures in support of patient autonomy, informed consent, respect for privacy and confidentiality, and the like. Trustees should ensure that hospital practice includes the patient, and when appropriate the family, as a partner in decision making about health care and medical treatment.

This principle enjoins trustees to take steps to ensure that limited hospital resources and services are utilized efficiently and effectively. When difficult distributive decisions must be made, they should be handled in a just and equitable fashion so that the quality of care is not substantially compromised and so that the effects of such decisions do not fall unfairly or disproportionately on the most vulnerable or the poorest patients.

Service to the community. Throughout American history, hospitals have been understood as civic institutions. They are not only places where individuals receive care or high-quality professional medicine is practiced; they are also resources dedicated to improving the public health and quality of civic life of the community as a whole. The health services hospitals provide are integral components of a community's identity and traditions. Trustees do well when they bear in mind the interconnection between what goes on inside the hospital and what occurs in the community outside.

The principle of service to the community recognizes this dimension of the trustee's role and the hospital's mission: *Trustees should govern hospital policy and deploy hospital resources in ways that enhance the health and quality of life in the broader community that the hospital serves.*

The mission of the hospital cannot be successfully pursued in isolation from the nature and quality of the surrounding community. Service to patients and families neither begins when the patient enters the hospital nor ends when he or she is discharged. This is one area where the scope of ethical responsibility is considerably broader than that of legal responsibility or liability.

Emergency rescue and acute stabilization are only the tips of the iceberg of health care needs in today's society. Chronic illness and disability, behaviorally related health risks, community mental health services, and the provision of adequate housing, nutrition, and support systems, both familial and profession-al, are the keys to serving the needs and rights of patients in the broader con-text of their lives. It makes little sense to repeatedly treat the individual symptoms of problems that are at root civic and systemic in nature.

Hospitals alone cannot cure civic or community problems, and in today's health economy they are sometimes hard pressed to attend even to the acute and emergency care responsibilities. But ethically responsible trusteeship requires a willingness to participate with other civic leaders in the search for broader community enhancement and civic renewal efforts.

A hospital—least of all a not-for-profit hospital—is not simply a business that sells something to the community out of self-interest. Neither is a hospital designed to give something to the community out of voluntary charity—even if it is a not-for-profit hospital. A hospital may indeed sometimes function like a business, and sometimes it will be called upon to be a charity, but above all it is a civic institution. It takes cognizance of the quality of civic life in the broader community because its very essence as an institution is at stake in efforts to promote public health and its participation with other community institutions in the ongoing task of civic preservation and renewal.

Institutional stewardship. Most trustees would agree with the emphasis we have placed on patient service and service to the broader community. They might not call these issues matters of "ethics," but they do acknowledge the norm and the sense of responsibility nonetheless. They recognize even more readily, however, their role in hospital governance and institutional steward-ship, responsibility, and leadership.

Hence the principle of institutional stewardship: *Trustees should sustain and enhance the integrity of the hospital as an institution, as an effective organization for the delivery of high quality health care services, and as a moral community of caregiving.*

Trustees are entrusted with the hospital's mission, but in practical terms that translates into working with the executive management of the facility to ensure that it is well run, fiscally sound, and professionally competent. In short, trustees must protect the interests of all parties who rely on the hospital or are significantly affected by its activities, in addition to protecting the hospital's financial assets and its license and accreditation.

Each of these duties is vital and ethically significant, and they form a part of what is meant by institutional stewardship. But the principle we formulate here is intended to go beyond these standard and well-recognized fiduciary obligations and to encompass the notion that ethical trusteeship is responsible for the maintenance and flourishing of the hospital's ethical integrity as an institution. Trustees are not entrusted simply with the governance of the hospital as an "asset," as a property with a certain market value. They are also—and no less significantly—entrusted with the care of the hospital as a vibrant and viable social and cultural system, a moral community comprised of many individuals from varied backgrounds with diverse needs, skills, and contributions to make to the whole.

Of course, this does not mean that a hospital should never be closed and its monetary value liquidated or converted to another socially beneficial use. Some hospitals have outlived their mission and their usefulness in a particular community; others, through mismanagement, the departure of key personnel, or lack of resources, have lost the ability to provide an adequate and competent level of service to their patients and the community. The responsibility of trustees to perceive when a hospital is no longer viable is as important as the responsibility to fight to ensure the hospital's viability and survival.

Fulfilling this principle requires certain kinds of conduct by individual trustees, certain kinds of conduct by the board of trustees collectively, and support for certain kinds of governance, administrative, and clinical policies and practices throughout the hospital. Here the general orientation offered by principles meets the more specific duties that trustees should fulfill when making particular decisions and taking action. And the ethical perspective on trustees as individuals meets the issue of the proper organization and functioning of the board as a collective decision-making system through which individual trustees exercise their own ethical responsibilities. The principle of institutional stewardship closes the circle on this relationship, so to speak. It reminds trustees that, even as the proper functioning of the board (and of the hospital as a whole) enables them to fulfill their duties, each individual trustee also has a duty to help create and sustain a well-functioning board.

THE ORGANIZATION OF THIS BOOK

There are many ways in which the essays in this volume could have been grouped and presented, for they deal with cross-cutting themes and issues.

Because they were developed in the context of a series of project meetings, they often play off against one another. The order of presentation we finally chose is based upon a rough distinction among contextual studies; philosophical, conceptual, and theoretical studies; and studies that address specific domains or particular problems within the contemporary hospital setting and its governance.

But these divisions of the book are rough and heuristic guides only. Many of the chapters in part II are in fact quite concrete and practically oriented, whereas the chapters in parts I and III each has a philosophical and theoretical underpinning of a certain kind. The normative and the descriptive, the ideal and the real, value and fact, ought and is—each of these intertwine in the chapters of this book as they do in the practice and decision making of individual hospital trustees and boards.

During the course of our project research, Bradford Gray, Linda Weiss, and other colleagues from the New York Academy of Medicine conducted a set of approximately 100 interviews with trustees and hospital chief executive officers in the New York metropolitan area, and six other hospitals that had considered sale to a for-profit purchaser. The findings from those interviews are presented in chapters 5 and 10. These chapters probe trustees' own conceptions of "ethics" and their own languages of self-description and self-understanding about the roles they play and the responsibilities they bear. They also show the kinds of questions trustees consider when they must make fundamental decisions about affiliation or merger with another institution, about the closing or reduction of particular hospital services, and about patient safety and quality-of-care issues within the hospital, among other issues.

Taking trustee ethics seriously does not require that all trustees must always agree. There is room within the scope of conscientious, ethical board service for a broad range of disagreement over many financial, institutional, and public policy issues that affect hospital operations today. Nonetheless, many trustees today feel buffeted by conflicting forces and are seeking to place such debates and policy disputes within some ethical context and perspective.

Some may be concerned that raising trustee awareness regarding ethics will lead trustees to seek more influence in the governance of their organizations at the expense of management. Again, the ethical perspective we offer does not stipulate any particular style or arrangement in the governance and management of hospitals. There is a spectrum of different working arrangements between boards and executives that permit each side to fulfill its functions responsibly and to discharge the ethical obligations of its respective roles.

The vision of ethics we offer here calls for a thoughtful, well-informed trustee, one who is not intrusive or overbearing in dealings with management, but who works as an effective partner with management and who prepares himself or herself to exercise responsibilities effectively and with sound reasoning and judgment. Careful discussion of ethics among trustees can assist in this regard, and in this way will also be beneficial to hospital management.

NOTES

1. Mary R. Anderlik, *The Ethics of Managed Care* (Bloomington: Indiana University Press, 2001).

2. We follow conventional usage in referring to the members of the governing board of not-for-profit organizations as "trustees" instead of "directors," which is used in the for-profit sector. Moreover, when we use the term "trustee" in this report, we refer not to trustees of not-for-profit organizations in general but specifically to a trustee of a not-for-profit hospital.

3. Bruce Jennings, Bradford H. Gray, Virginia A. Sharpe, Linda Weiss, and Alan R. Fleischman, "Ethics and Trusteeship for Health Care: Hospital Board Service in Turbulent Times," *Hastings Center Report (Special Supplement)* 32, no. 4 (July–August 2002): S1–S28.

4. For a more detailed discussion of the ethical framework sketched below, see Jennings et al., "Ethics and Trusteeship for Health Care," S14–S16.

5. Harvey J. Goldschmid, "The Fiduciary Duties of Nonprofit Directors and Officers: Paradoxes, Problems, and Proposed Reforms," *Journal of Corporation Law* 23, no. 4 (summer 1998).

6. David H. Smith, *Entrusted: The Moral Responsibilities of Trusteeship* (Bloomington: Indiana University Press, 1995).

PART I

Hospital Trusteeship in Legal and Social Context

THE TRUSTEES' DILEMMA

Hospitals as Benevolence or Business—
Looking Back a Century

Elizabeth Robilotti and David Rosner

THE HOSPITAL IN TRANSITION

I n 1920, just after the end of World War I, the fledgling journal *Hospital Management*, the publication of the newly organized American Hospital Association, published a frontispiece illustration depicting a hospital superintendent referring to a book titled *Industrial Efficiency* (figure 1.1).[1] With reports and charts cluttering the administrator's desk, and with a wastebasket piled high with crumpled pages, the illustration told the reader that it was now time for the new hospital to begin "Borrowing a Volume from Industry." The message was clear: Now was the time for trustees and administrators to rethink the meaning, organization, and purpose of the hospital. Modern management was a key to the hospital's future success, and the magazine *Hospital Management*, "Published in the Interest of Executives in Every Department of Hospital Work," would play a prominent role. The older charity hospital, long the provider of medical and social services to poor people, had fostered bad management habits among administrators and trustees whose hearts were said to have overwhelmed their judgment. Now the entire administration, organization, architecture, and financial underpinnings of the institution had to be rethought.

This call for new principles in organizing the hospital reflected profound changes in the social function of the hospital during the previous twenty years. The traditional understanding of the hospital was increasingly challenged by the changing medical needs of patients and shifting demands forced upon it by private practitioners and administrators reared in a different tradition and a different social world. Older charity hospitals, most founded in the late nineteenth century, had served specific ethnic and religious communities in ways that were now coming under scrutiny. These older institutions satisfied a full range of purposes from social service, to medical care, to moral reform. Patients entered the institutions for a variety of reasons, only some of them medical. During economic depressions, hospital censuses ballooned as unemployed single workers, both male and female, suffering from a variety of vague, often common, complaints would enter the hospital. Single girls, pregnant out of wedlock and unable to remain at home or in their communities, would seek refuge in lying-in hospitals awaiting the birth of their child. Children, deemed abandoned or abused, would be brought to the foundling or children's hospitals where they received the care of deaconesses, nuns, or other personnel. Care was intimately linked to restoring social and moral well-being as well as physical health.

The moral and social objectives of these diverse nineteenth-century institutions had a profound impact on their internal order and organization. Most significantly, charity hospitals often functioned more like homes than as acute care facilities. Patients stayed for months and sometimes years, as their moral and physical ills were tended to. In lying-in hospitals, women were required to see their children through nursing or, if the child died at birth or in infancy, to nurse the children of other mothers who had died. In children's hospitals, administrators often limited visiting privileges for parents to a brief period on Sunday afternoons for fear that they might provide poor examples to the children under the hospital's care. Trustees often held a religious conception of suffering that they believed required as much attention as the physiological ailments. For the trustees, ward patients invoked an urge to care, especially by their "appropriately Christian and deferential version of suffering."[2] Patients lived in the "house" along with physicians, nurses, and other staff, and were seen as "residents" or "inmates" who had responsibilities as part of this extended family. Out of bed for much of their months'-long stays, patients learned the moral lessons that trustees and administrators sought to impart about the moral value of work, the need to care for one's brethren, and the righteous ways to live, all of which were intrinsic to any meaningful cure of disease. In this era, ideas about bacteriology were intermingled with older moral notions of disease as a form of divine retribution, moral suasion, good food, and education in the ways of a moral life. Other forms of social education were as important as the unproven claims of physicians or bacteriologists whose belief in the germ as a cause of illness was still largely unproven and untested.

In general, the use of large, undifferentiated wards with many beds—the usual form of housing in the nineteenth century hospital—met the needs of an institution trying to supervise and control patients confined for long periods of time. First, the ward, with beds lined along its walls, allowed nurses or attendants to watch many patients simultaneously and guaranteed the strict supervision of potentially disruptive or untrustworthy poorer "inmates." Second, the ward arrangement allowed patients to socialize in an institution that in practice substituted for the home. Third, patients who were ambulatory could learn good work habits by serving as orderlies and nurses and by helping those other patients near at hand who were incapable of helping themselves.

In being dominated by lay trustees, these charity hospitals exemplified an elite's awareness of their stewardship responsibilities to the poor and destitute segments of society.[3] From 1860 to 1900, rapid urbanization and immigration sparked the development of hospitals more for humanitarian reasons than out of scientific necessity, and this led lay trustees into conflict with physicians over the best manner for operating the hospital. For instance, a variety of subcommittees, the ranks of which were derived from the hospital trustees, dictated different aspects of hospital service and acted as the admissions committee for ward patients.[4] Potential patients either applied to a trustee they knew, or offered a letter from a clergyman attesting to their moral character. The "truly worthy," those patients who were temporarily down on their luck or who had swayed from the righteous path through "no fault of their own," were allowed into the charity institutions. The "unworthy poor," those who were thought to be unreachable by the techniques or message the charity institution sought to convey, were denied admittance.

It is no accident that many of the charity institutions, particularly on the East Coast and Midwest, were closely affiliated with particular ethnic and religious groups. The vast majority were organized during periods of massive immigration from eastern and southern European groups. In New York City, for example, the hospitals named Saint Vincent's, Jew's (later Mount Sinai), French, German (later Lenox Hill), Saint Luke's, and Presbyterian all grew out of the growing sense of disorder that affected American cities as literally millions of poor, non-English-speaking Catholics and Jews flooded into American ports.

Trustee conceptions of benevolence influenced the method of patient care within the late-nineteenth-century institution. The only social characteristics that were used to separate patients in wards were sex, age, and medical condition. Although the institutions were often administered by specific religious or sectarian orders, most trustees believed in a moral obligation to admit poorer patients regardless of race or religion. In fact, given their strong missionary zeal, many trustees understood the inclusion of a wide range of religious, racial, and ethnic groups to be an important indication of the usefulness of the institution.[5] Every year the annual reports of the various hospitals remarked on the wide variety of races, religions, and nationalities that appeared in their beds. Even the architectural detail of many of these institutions reflected the overriding concern with its social and moral objectives, with many of them built to resemble churches, mansions, and homes rather than prisons, schools, or factories.

THE NEW MANAGEMENT

In the years following World War I, the changing social and cultural structure of the United States left hospital trustees confounded about the future of their institutions. Trustees, mired in debates about the impact of changing economic conditions on their charitable missions and daily operations, were forced to address the new trends of capitalism, consumerism, and standardized production. As captains of industry introduced ordered production models into American business, scientific management's aphorisms of standardization and efficiency filled boardrooms throughout the county. Hospital trustees watching the efficiency tidal wave wash over American business were not immune to its influences, even within the walls of their sturdily constructed hospitals. Whether or not hospitals, trustees, and their staffs would succumb to scientific management's influence and call into question the ideological foundations of the hospital would be debated throughout the 1920s.

New conceptions of management and the changing role of the hospital were also reflected in the changing mission and ranks of the American Hospital Association. It had originally been founded at the turn of the century as the Association of Hospital Superintendents, a grouping of hospital superintendents interested in exchanging operational information. Now, the association changed its mission and membership requirements to reflect the new pressures on hospitals. It expanded its membership to include assistant superintendents and other junior staff, and it officially changed its name to the American Hospital Association. In 1907, the goal of the organization changed from creating a forum for dialogue about charity hospitals to being a vehicle for "the promotion of economy and efficiency in hospital management."[6] More than just a change in semantics, this new goal foreshadowed the debates that would be played out in *Hospital Management* and in the association's affiliated institutions for the rest of the twentieth century.

The dilemma faced by trustees about how to run a charity institution while adopting Progressive Era business practices plagued the heads of charity institutions. One cover of *Hospital Management*, echoing the new interest in efficiency, depicted a hospital superintendent manning the employment office window (figure 1.2). On the wall, the "help wanted" sign lists the available positions, ranging from dishwashers and maids to cooks and laundry workers. The superintendent remarks to a robotic applicant, "You look efficient. You're hired."[7] The new hire, a "labor-saver," could perform multiple tasks, making him a "popular employee." This cover, appearing in 1918, not only highlighted the shift toward efficiency but also reflected other issues confronted by hospitals, especially regarding employment and employee loyalty.

Notions of scientific management challenged the cultural identity of quirky charity hospitals as trustees were forced to reconcile notions of efficiency with traditional charitable missions. An earlier *Hospital Management* cover showed the erosion of the old paternalistic relationship between hospital superintendents and the hospital labor force.[8] This 1917 illustration (figure 1.3) shows "Mother Hubbard," an old female superintendent with a small purse and a huge empty food basket, evicting a throng of workers from a giant shoe, the hospital dormitory, telling the downcast workers "the cupboard was bare." No longer should the hospital be considered the "house" or home where staff, other than young doctors in training and nurses, would be given living accommodations. Such paternalistic practices were presented as a leftover from an earlier era.

Hospital Management, with its targeted readership of trustees, hospital managers, and administrators, chronicled concerns about the consequences of a loss of charitable mission and hospital identity. This theme—that the hospital administrator had to begin running his or her institution like any other big business—recurred over and over again in the pages of the new journal in its early years of publication. The journal sought to transform the older, paternalistic hospital, long governed by a set of moral, social, and charitable principles, into a "modern" institution, freed from the economic, organizational, and ideological constraints that had limited its effectiveness in the emerging era of modern medicine. The magazine promoted the methods of management that had transformed a rural, agricultural society into one of the leading economic engines on earth.

Hospital Management noted trustee fears about standardized factory model hospitals in an illustration titled "The Hospital Production Sheet" (figure 1.4).[9] In this illustration, the trustee, hospital superintendent, and doctor—cognizant of the changing climate of business and employment relationships occurring within American society—struggle to reconcile the differences between hospital and factory output. Whereas the factory produced such easily quantifiable products as motors and transmissions, the hospital's outputs, measured in diagnoses and deaths, were impossible to describe with simple numerical measurements. This illustration reflects many of the concerns voiced by trustees and administrators that the factory-efficiency model drew the hospital away from what should be its primary mission, the care of patients.

The hospital was not a machine shop, a production line, or a mechanical operation in which machines, or people who acted like machines, produced widgets. Rather, the hospital was an intensely human-driven institution, overwhelmingly staffed by people whose ideological commitment to helping, caring, and charity often provided them with reason to accept low wages, long hours, and sometimes horrifying working and living conditions. Caritas, not carrots, was the incentives to treat dying patients, poverty-stricken dependent people, the sick, and the infirm.

For trustees, who were often the moral as well as commercial leaders of ethnic and religious communities, the idea of transforming their institution using tools and concepts borrowed from commercial operations was anything but obvious; many had joined the boards of the institutions primarily because they were charitable, social agencies. They feared such a transformation could undercut the very foundations of what made the hospital run. It could also undermine their own role as moral guardians of poor people and their own service-oriented justification for becoming trustees. What was the hospital in modern American life? What values, purposes, and ideals should inform its staff and administrators? What was the role of the trustee, once the overseer of the moral as well as medical role of the institution, to become as the hospital modernized and transformed itself into a new kind of institution? The journal *Hospital Management*, which had the motto "Published in the Interest of Executives in Every Department of Hospital Work," confronted these questions head-on.

Ambivalent Trusteeship

While the journal *Hospital Management's* purpose was to be the unambiguous promoter of the business-oriented hospital organization, in fact the journal's illustrations generally showed great ambivalence about the new direction the American Hospital Association was promoting. After all, the implicit point of the illustrations was that there were deep problems imbedded in transforming an institution from a charity into an industrial model. Would the underlying moral purpose of the facility be destroyed by such a change in course? Would a staff, working for wages, treated like workers rather than as coparticipants in a great moral undertaking, rebel, or resign? In a period of tremendous labor unrest, could a hospital maintain its underlying moral rationale while adopting measures seen as antilabor? Would the broader community outside the hospital accept and support an institution that defined itself as a machine shop, measuring its success in raw numbers rather than humanitarian outputs? Indeed, would wealthy and prominent community leaders be drawn to contribute to an institution or participate on the board of a hospital if the institution went too far in reshaping its moral mission into something they could not understand? With competing benevolent institutions like colleges and universities seeking to attract donations themselves, how could the hospital position itself so that it could benefit from its charitable image yet move into a new century freed from the monetary and organizational constraints of its nineteenth-century origins?

Questions about the effect on care of the new efficiency models dominated the cover of *Hospital Management*. The magazine presented illustrations depicting exaggerated scenarios of the hospital in its transition to a modern institution. For example, one cover shows a superintendent, sweat pouring down his face, pleading with a line of nurses to attend to an emergency case (figure 1.5). The nurse running to the end of the time-clock line replies, "Just a minute. I've got to fall in line and punch the clock." The caption above reads, "Will it come to this?" This illustration demonstrates administrator concerns about industrial infiltration of hospital operations. Ironically, the social relations that allowed charitable institutions to function cheaply could too easily be disrupted if the ideological chemistry of the old charity hospital changed too dramatically. Oddly, the very goal of efficiency would destroy the low-cost facility, and false notions of efficiency could all too easily outweigh emergency in importance in new industrial hospital models. The illustration reinforces this fear, as a notice from the "factory inspector" hangs ominously above the line of nurses reinforcing the newly instituted labor regulations.

For most of the nineteenth century, the charity hospitals of the country were inexpensive institutions that could run on relatively small sums of money each year. The minimal technical abilities of hospitals in the late nineteenth century, along with a patient-derived workforce, kept yearly operating budgets at most institutions low, in the range of $30,000–$35,000. These hospitals—funded by the institutions' benefactors, a variety of state and local government sources, and a minimal amount of patient payments—ran at modest deficits every year, deficits that were generally covered by fund-raising events or end-of-the-year trustee contributions.

By the end of the century, however, the cost for patient care began to increase substantially as advances in medical technology and changing standards of cleanliness began to affect the care provided. Also, as philanthropists faced competing demands from other agencies and as the number of poor people seeking services increased substantially, hospitals found themselves strapped for funds. Increasingly, hospital trustees were forced to make hard choices about the future of their charitable enterprises, and they began to turn to new and untested sources of income: private middle-class patients.

Hence, trustees were both attracted and frightened by the calls for greater efficiency, the transformation of their institutions into medical facilities, and the reorganization of services. On the one hand, new technologies like the X-ray, the autoclave, and sterile or antiseptic surgical rooms, along with new amenities, better food, and a larger staff, were raising the cost of an institution that had previously been low technology and highly labor intensive, and yet very cheap to run. On the other hand, altering the purpose of the institution meant introducing new patients who were attracted to the facility for medical, not social, reasons. This, in turn, meant that a subtle power shift could easily occur in the new hospital as authority shifted to physicians and those affiliated with the new science of medicine and away from the trustees who were associated with the model of hospital care based on moral and social reform.

In a *Hospital Management* illustration titled "The Class in Hospital Designing," the resistance of trustees to the new efficiency model is reflected in the fact that trustees, superintendents, and other staff are all infantilized, forced to sit in a classroom and instructed by "the public" who tells them their ideas of hospital design are outmoded (figure 1.6). Fewer and fewer people were receiving care at home; the hospital must adapt to increased patient admissions by restructuring their facility. In the illustration, "the public" tells trustees that semiprivate and private rooms rather than charity wards were the future.[10] According to *Hospital Management*, wages were high, charity wards were unfilled, and revenue from private-ward patients would stabilize the hospital's finances. The implication was both clear and threatening: Hospital administrators in the beginning of the twentieth century had to think about competing for paying patients, in part by remodeling or even rebuilding their institutions.

THE CONSEQUENCES OF A MIDDLE-CLASS CLIENTELE

The consequences of the introduction of paying patients were numerous for hospital trustees and superintendents. First, paying patients demanded new amenities never even considered in the charity institution. The middle class, formerly served at home by a staff of private practitioners, private duty nurses, and servants, would never come to an institution designed for poor people. Hospitals would be forced to construct new facilities or reorganize existing facilities to accommodate the new demands. In addition, the marketplace, not the social service department or the ambulance, would determine where paying patients would end up. Competition for paying patients among the institutions in a city marked a significant departure for hospitals that previously had a guaranteed patient population drawn from the ethnic and religious communities that had sponsored their foundation in the first place. Paying patients would be looking for amenities and medical prestige, not protection from the cold.

The trustees' own legitimacy would be brought into question as they lost their role as stewards for the lower classes and as overseers of decisions about the moral worthiness of the patient population. In the old paternalistic hospital, patients could not simply turn to their physicians to gain admittance to a hospital. In fact, few physicians had hospital "privileges" in the charity institution. Rather, a sponsor, a prominent community member like a wealthy merchant or minister, would write a letter to the lay trustee of the hospital attesting to their moral worthiness, and by implication to their stable lower-class position within the community. With significant exceptions of accident cases, travelers, or visitors to the community who might bypass the scrutiny of the trustees by entering the hospital through the emergency room, the charity hospital carefully selected those to whom it would extend its charity services.[11] Now trustees were faced by the possibility of losing control over the day-to-day administration of the hospital as administrators saw that the physician, not the trustee, largely controlled whom the institution did and did not serve. Further, the patients themselves would see the physicians, rather than the trustees, as the significant authorities in the new hospital.

A frontispiece illustration in *Hospital Management* reflected the dilemmas facing trustees and administrators as the language of standardization and efficiency was introduced into the lexicon of the hospital administrator and trustee. In one, a man representing "the public" balances a scale with the "standardized hospital" complete with labs, an X-ray department, and operating facilities on one side, and the patient in a wheelchair on the other (figure 1.7).[12] The hospital building, resembling a multistoried department store rather than a house or religious institution, was a conglomeration of individual departments and services. With regard to the fact that the building is devoid of the individual character and moral overtones of earlier hospital architecture, the "public" asks at what point does the drive to create the new institution conflict with its historical mission of caring for people?

In another illustration, the female hospital superintendent mournfully faces a desk full of bills for food, surgical supplies, and fuel, while a child, with a suit labeled "hospital rates," stands by (figure 1.8).[13] The child, obviously representing the patient, asks, "Mother, don't you think I need a new suit?" The piles of bills represent all the new services available at the hospital, from laundry to surgical services. The old female superintendent is reluctant to increase hospital rates, for that seems like an abandonment of her charitable mission. However, the hospital rates suit simply cannot cover the child, who is stamped "increased operating expenses." New ideas and an abandonment of the older charitable model was inevitable, despite the misgivings of the superintendent.

From Female to Male Care

The reorganization of the hospital also changed the composition of the workforce. Not only did professionals replace patient workers, but the traditionally female roles of hospital superintendents were replaced by male administrators. Although the public image of the institution was that of a social service, women began to complain of the preference that trustees in the early decades of the twentieth century showed for males interested in becoming head administrators.

In the years when the health system grew dramatically, hospital and clinic administration was seen as the natural preserve of largely single middle-class women whose social role was to maintain the harmony, stability, and cohesiveness of their communities. Just as the married woman ran the household, single women—often sisters in Catholic institutions or nurses and laywomen in smaller ethnic facilities—were appropriate candidates to run the community's voluntary institutions.[14] In these generally smaller institutions, they were responsible for both the caring and business functions of the facility. As late as 1928, one woman administrator noted that "a hospital superintendent should have a working knowledge of business methods. I am confident that many hospitals need and want as superintendent women who have health, business ability and some understanding of medical and nursing problems."[15] For most of the first third of the century, caring and financial stewardship were considered to be equally necessary for the hospital administrator. Women, therefore, with their claim on the household and emotional lives of the community, made excellent candidates for administrative positions.

Women's role as protectors of the moral life of the family added a degree of legitimacy to their positions as hospital administrators. In the urban society of the late nineteenth and early twentieth centuries, where dependence, poverty, and illness were often interpreted as interlocking indications of the general morality—or immorality—of patients, medical cure was seen as intimately linked to the success of moral reform within the institution. Hence the administrator, as the person responsible for the institution, largely controlled the program that would teach patients acceptable standards of moral behavior. Internally, facilities reflected the underlying moral goals of the originators and the head administrator. The superintendent was responsible for the daily management of the institution and functioned as the patriarch or matriarch of the extended family that the hospital was supposed to resemble.

The redefinition of the hospital administrator reflected a fundamental change in the underlying political economy of the institution. Between the late 1890s and the advent of the Great Depression, the institution changed its mission, revamped its services, and altered its financial base. By the 1920s, the institution was reorganizing in response to the new needs of potential customers, and the basis for the maternalist female administrator faded. "There has . . . been great injustice shown toward the woman executive," complained one hospital administrator from Pennsylvania. "A woman builds upon a substantial foundation but when the institution has expanded in its capacity for increased service, in its popularity with the public, in its wholesome influence upon the community, the question seems to be raised in the minds of [these trustees], should we not pass on to a man's control, and this often when a woman has mortgaged her health in her impassioned service to the institution."[16]

What this administrator illustrated was the deeply rooted and then-developing strains on the health system. In her statement, she was not just bemoaning the passing of a career track from females to males. She was also noting a transformation of her institution from one that was community and family based to one that was managed by people with little connection to its charitable origins. She worried about the uneasy alliance between health care and business. In the view of many, the new vision of the institution and its administrators lacked the strong and coherent ideology of the older charity institution. The 1920s marked the beginning of a period of turmoil within hospital administration.

The traditional association of the hospital with charity care gave the institution a clear class-identification that trustees were eager to abandon, and the movement of men into administration signaled an important change in the social structure and mission of the institution. This shift in gender helped trustees in their efforts to begin the process of cleansing their institutions of the class-bound identification of a charity facility. Furthermore, as medicine became a more accepted justification of a hospital's function and as physicians became more integral to the financial and service structure of these institutions, trustees sought persons whose identity was more intimately associated with medicine rather than charity. Trustees sought individuals who could identify for them potential problems associated with the medicalization of the institution and its business interests. Hence, when able, trustees turned to physicians to administer their institutions. By 1929, fully 37 percent of all administrators were male physicians. In teaching hospitals, the percentage was even higher, hovering around 53 percent.[17]

FROM CHARITY CARE TO MEDICAL CARE

The older role of the hospital as charity was undermined by a new rationale for the institution based upon medical rather than charitable intent. Hospitals, emerging as the workshops of physicians, became primarily scientific institutions grafted onto social service facilities. As hospitals increasingly sought to attract patients from the middle or upper classes of society, they sought to build services with more amenities and greater comforts than had previously been necessary in the charity institution. Private and semiprivate wards began to replace the charity ward; and private wings and private nursing were introduced into facilities that previously had made few if any class distinctions regarding patients. Similarly, visiting medical personnel came to be ubiquitous in institutions where, only a few decades before, few physicians were permitted into the wards on any regular basis.

The medical profession was in the midst of its own reorganization at the end of the nineteenth century, and this dramatically challenged the primacy of the trustee as the leader of the hospital. Nineteenth-century American medicine was characterized by floundering empiricism. Although trial and error was responsible for the few pharmacological discoveries up to that point, this process was slow to advance medical science. In addition, medical practitioners were divided into a variety of conceptual camps, complicating the standardization of American medicine. Throughout much of the nineteenth century, the disparate demands of different groups in different areas of the country created a diverse body of therapeutic knowledge and practice. Accordingly, training differed for rural practitioners, urban practitioners, homeopaths, allopaths, eclectics, Thomsonians, and the host of other practitioners of the "art" of medicine. Even those treating different classes and ethnic groups within the population were forced by the realities of the medical marketplace to adjust their practice.

The lack of a universal ideology in the theory and practice of medicine presented numerous challenges to advancing medical science. Throughout the late nineteenth century, the only thing consistent about medicine in America was its inconsistency. This disparity was reflected in the differences between medical nosologies, views, and theoretical positions. Different groups of practitioners generally identified with differing "schools" or "sects" of medicine. Rural areas produced a wide variety of practitioners who depended mostly on herbal treatments. Thomsonians and later eclectics were among the various botanical schools that developed throughout rural New England, the South, and the Midwest. Generally, these groups incorporated local folk custom into their therapeutics. In urban areas, regular practitioners, homeopaths, and a host of others with differing medical viewpoints and practices competed strongly with each other for the patronage of patients.[18] Across the country, the quality of medical education varied enormously. Institutions ranged from medical colleges, such as at Harvard University, the University of Pennsylvania, and Physicians and Surgeons (later Columbia University), with minimal entrance requirements, through proprietary medical schools operated for a fee by physicians looking to supplement their incomes, to loosely regulated apprenticeships.

Proprietary schools impeded the systematization of American medical education. The broad range of teaching standards further complicated standardization efforts at the end of the nineteenth century. The proprietary facilities produced physicians of limited experience who were challenged by an emerging contingent of scientifically focused practitioners. These proponents of scientific medicine operated out of universities, medical schools, and hospitals.

While these university medical men apprised themselves of advances in European medical science and techniques, the proprietary physicians remained committed to only local remedies. A rift developed between the university physicians, who spearheaded the movement to reform medical education on a "scientific" basis, and local practitioners, who favored their parochial remedies.

This ideological conflict translated into a competition for patients as the overabundance of medical practitioners persisted through the end of the nineteenth century. Medicine in the nineteenth century lacked any basis for claiming authority, because most medical techniques were ineffective. However, the bacteriological revolution of the 1870s and the development of antiseptic surgery after 1880 helped medicine transform itself into an organization of "unparalleled professional power." Through these efforts, medicine hoped to eliminate the quackery and sectarianism that had proliferated throughout the nineteenth century, and to establish a scientific basis for medicine.[19]

The relationship between doctors and patients was not necessarily the product of a deep-seated intellectual or professional belief in democracy, nor the importance of trust and understanding in the therapeutic process. Rather, it was in large measure an outgrowth of the professional environment where practitioners, working in an era of significant medical uncertainty with regard to procedures and outcomes, were in severe competition with each other for clients. The uncertainty of medical practice contributed to the reluctance of the trustee to let medical students have access to patients. In hanging onto some semblance of their charity mission, trustees were reluctant to relinquish patient control to practitioners and their students, whom they considered unregulated and unpracticed. However, trustee clinical authority withered throughout the beginning of the twentieth century as physicians greatly increased their influence over hospital admissions.

The difficulty created by this lack of uniformity was further complicated by the explosive growth of the most unregulated forms of medical education, the independent "medical schools" during the nineteenth century. More than four hundred medical schools were established between 1800 and 1900, dramatically increasing the disparity of medical education in America. The proprietary facilities churned out poorly trained physicians at a stupendous rate. This resulted in an oversupply of physicians of varying quality.

In the decades surrounding the turn of the century, a significant reform movement arose within medicine itself that held as its guiding principles the need to standardize medical education. Underlying this reform effort lay the notion that by standardizing the training of physicians and by controlling entry into the profession through licensure, medical practice itself would become more uniform. The movement culminated in the now-classic Carnegie Bulletin Number Four, the "Flexner Report," that called for the reorganization of the medical school curriculum.

The Flexner Report was an end product of a long and tortured movement among medical educators, predominantly within the American Medical Association's Council on Medical Education, to standardize American medicine. But it was only successful in certain narrow respects. Although medical practice would remain a field filled with medical uncertainty and nonstandardized procedures performed by individual practitioners, the standardization of the social background of medical practitioners would be achieved. By the end of the nineteenth century, the eclectic nature of medical practice and the largely unregulated environment in which medicine developed had created a large and diverse set of educational institutions that catered to women, blacks, and poor students. In fact, there were sixteen women's medical schools by 1900, and ten black medical colleges, primarily in the southern states, by the same year. Also, the majority of medical students attending the various proprietary medical colleges were lower or lower middle class in social background. But, by 1916, only one women's medical college and two black schools remained in existence, and many of the proprietary institutions that once catered to part-time and working students went out of existence.

Reformers of medical education saw little need to ensure the social diversity of practitioners. In part, they thought that the growing trend toward scientifically based medicine would eradicate the need for schools directed at particular social groups. Instead, many reformers believed that standardized requirements would level the playing field for medical school admissions. Short of achieving equality though standardization, many proponents of the Flexner Report believed that medicine rooted in the principles of science would make social diversity among medical practitioners unnecessary.

Increasingly, standardized medical practice infiltrated hospital clinical procedures. As *Hospital Management* demonstrated in the cover illustration of "Mother Hubbard" evicting the hospital labor force, physicians at the turn of the century gained greater access to patients, even becoming the only residential laborers at the hospital (figure 1.3).[20] This increased access to patients troubled many older paternalistic trustees who were accustomed to having a supervisory role over patient admission and care. Scientific medicine made trustee involvement in the provision of care unnecessary. The new standardized model of American medicine further distanced paternalistic trustees from hospital patients and again brought into question the sustainability of a charitable mission.

THE ASSAULT ON TRUSTEES

With new advances in medicine came an increase in physician private practice. In an era of increasing operating costs and harsh competition for paying patients, the medical profession gained new influence within the walls of the trustees' hospital. The assault on trustee authority was not only waged by physicians, but by the ever-increasing number of disciplines associated with standardized scientific medical care. With a cover titled "The New Member of the 'Team,'" *Hospital Management* reflected the trends in hospital treatment (figure 1.9).[21] The old model of a trustee and a house staff physician walking the charity wards surveying patient progress had, by the 1920s, been replaced by new methods of standardized care. A "team" of providers made vital decisions regarding hospital operations. Included on the team were trustees, physicians, the superintendent, the superintendent of nurses, and the dietician. Though the trustee was still part of the committee, the trustee's exclusive control over patients had been destroyed by the coming standardization.

Although doctors had always played a role in caring for patients within the hospital, physicians' access to institutions caused tremendous antagonism with lay trustees. Trustees recognized the threat an "open" institution posed to their authority, one in which numerous physicians had access to the wards and patients. By opening up their institutions to private doctors, the trustees faced the danger of losing moral, medical, and cultural control of the institution. From the perspective of many upper-class trustees, local private practitioners understood nothing about the underlying moral and social rationale of the facility. Unlike the younger house staff that depended upon trustees for closely guarded learning experiences, private practitioners had little understanding of the larger goals of the institution and exhibited loyalty only to their private patients. From the perspective of the trustees, they brought with them a petty entrepreneurial focus and undermined the paternalism, communality, oversight, and structure of the hospital. For many institutions, however, concerns over the private practitioners missing a sense of charitable mission were tabled in the face of overwhelming economic necessity. Local practitioners entering the ranks of the hospital staff often brought with them a sizable private patient base, from which the hospital could generate much needed revenue.

Many trustees, faced with the challenges of opening their previously tightly guarded doors to local physicians while continuing to remain true to their charitable origins, settled these dichotomous goals by organizing two parallel structures of health service within the hospital. In part, the parallel structures were meant to protect the charity institution while providing the amenities demanded by a new, wealthier class of patient. In the process, however, the trustees institutionalized certain elements of two-class care by providing the charity patient with what they assumed was a more appropriate service and allowing the paying patient to be placed in the hands of the practitioners who the trustees generally saw as undereducated, crass, and ill prepared to care for most of their charity cases. Trustees sought to protect their charitable mission by restricting the outside physician to visiting privileges, rather than allowing them the advantages of full staff membership. By keeping the local practitioner out of the formal structure of the facility, trustees believed they could preserve the sanctity of their wards.

In addition, trustees revamped the physical structure of their hospitals to separate the charity cases from the paying patients. With these efforts, the trustees hoped to shield their charity charges from the commercial aspects of health care. Although private practice was to become an economic necessity in the voluntary hospital, it was not introduced by trustees solely to reward private practitioners and private patients. Rather, it was introduced in its particular way to protect charity patients—the true objective of the hospitals' mission—from an unaccountable and commercial private practice. Far from attempting to turn the institution into a "physician's workshop," many trustees sought to isolate private practice in private wings and to reap the economic benefits without jeopardizing their charity cases.

Hospital Management covers reflected trustee concerns about dealing with the changing hospital client base. These changes brought into question traditional charitable motives for everything from employee relationships to measuring the community benefit of the hospital. For example, as the hospital moved away from its altruistic roots and expelled the workforce from the hospital dormitories, it became difficult to recruit long-term workers. Trustees continued to worry that the standardized model of scientific medicine advocated by physicians and reformers could not meet the needs of patients.

Throughout the first half of the twentieth century, trustees were forced to confront the conflicts inherent in trying to run a modern hospital with administrative, intellectual, and economic tools borrowed from management. It was not clear that business and benevolence were natural allies in running an institution that was aimed at serving sick and dependent people in communities that were diverse and often disorganized. What the purpose of the trustee was and what he or she should be doing were obvious questions that needed to be addressed. Yet the paradox of the trustees' role was overwhelming. On the one hand, the trustee was often drawn from the business and commercial communities because of his or her wealth, prestige, or organizational acumen; on the other, the trustee generally came to the hospital because the institution had such dramatically different goals from the everyday world—goals that were clearly altruistic.

In general, the hospital was deeply imbedded with a culture and a history that was in stark conflict with the commercializing world of the twentieth century. Caught up in the industrial models popularized by proponents of scientific management, trustees opened their hospitals to infiltration by ideas and practices that often undermined the very goals they sought to promote. How to reconcile this conflict would plague trustees throughout the century.

At the beginning of the twenty-first century, hospital trustees face similar problems of balancing the mission to heal and provide charity service in an ever-evolving American economic and social structure dominated by the for-profit business model. Although the industrial model that confounded trustees and their charity missions at the beginning of the twentieth century is now rapidly shifting toward a global economic structure based on informational rather than industrial development, trustees are still providing the same complex product: health care. There are limits to the effectiveness of business-style cost cutting and organizational benefits when they are applied to the health care market. As one health care consultant explained, "These institutions are vastly more complicated than any business. You are literally custom making a product for everyone who comes in."[22] The complexities of running what has traditionally been a mission-oriented charity organization in an increasingly for-profit environment continues to plague trustees. Hospitals are no longer as poor as the charity patients they serve, and end-of-the-year debt is no longer a useful means of proving neediness to encourage donations.[23]

Contemporary hospitals are a mix of for-profit and not-for-profit institutions, where the bottom lines are watched as closely as the telemetry monitors.[24] Recent scandals and accusations of misplaced priorities have brought the entire hospital industry, and the for-profit hospital market in particular, under closer scrutiny. The government investigation of Columbia/HCA and the eventual overthrow of its mastermind, Richard Scott, is just one example of the perils facing for-profit hospitals.

Scott, realizing that hospitals operated in a quasi-industrial capital market with ready access to a "seemingly open spigot of government and private insurance money,"[25] decided to further push the limits of acceptable business practice in the health care market. He and Columbia/HCA sold shares of hospitals to the doctors serving the community and provided incentives to hospital executives who achieved certain financial benchmarks.[26] Scott developed a series of investor-owned institutions, operating under the dangerous philosophy that hospital profits and healthy patients went hand in hand.

However, as Gerard Anderson, director of the Johns Hopkins University Center for Hospital Finance and Management, has explained, such a system often left hospital trustees with an ethical dilemma—the same dilemma that trustees in the earlier twentieth century faced—how to balance the needs of patients with the profit motives of shareholders. Anderson continued, "In order to generate substantial profit margins, they [for-profit hospitals] need to take some liberties."[27] What these "liberties" are, however, is not at all clear. The traditional balance between the needs of patients and the needs of the institution has taken on a new persona. No longer is the balancing act between institutional efficiency and financial viability. Now, in more and more cases, the financial interests of investors far removed from patient care or even the institutions that they ostensibly own, affect the provision of hospital resources and quality of patient care. How does one condone taking "liberties" with people's lives merely for the pursuit of profit?

Vol. X, No. 5
November, 1920

HOSPITAL MANAGEMENT

417 S. Dearborn
Street,
Chicago

Published in the Interest of Executives in Every Department of Hospital Work

Borrowing a Volume from Industry

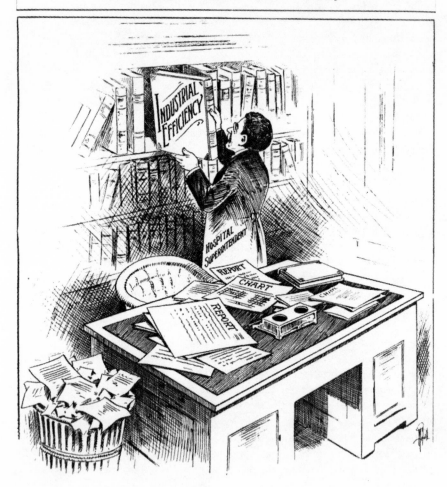

FIGURE 1.1.   A hospital superintendent referring to a book titled *Industrial Efficiency.*

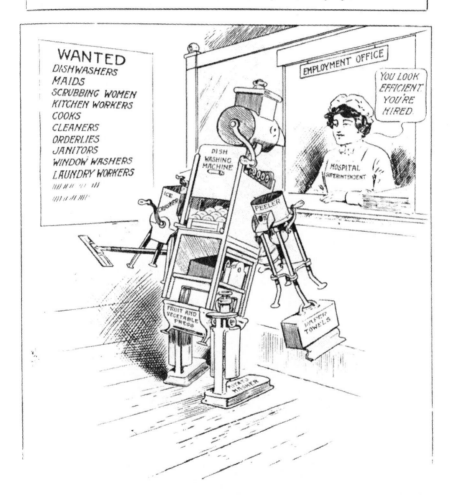

FIGURE 1.2.   Cover of *Hospital Management* depicting a hospital superintendent staffing the employment office window.

HOSPITAL MANAGEMENT

June, 1917
Vol. III, No. 5

608 S. Dearborn
Street,
Chicago

Published in the Interest of Executives in Every Department of Hospital Work

.ntered as second class matter May 14, 1917, at the post office at Chicago, Ill., under the act of March 3, 1879.

A Modern Version of The Old Woman Who Lived in a Shoe

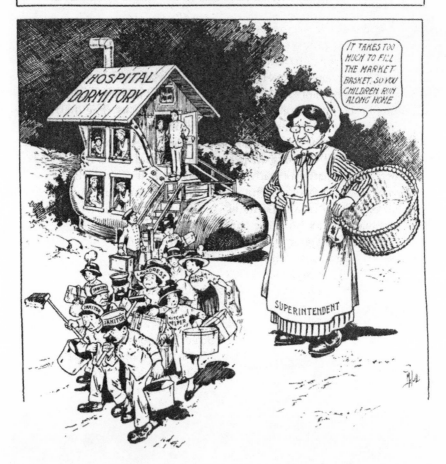

FIGURE 1.3.   Mother Hubbard evicting a throng of workers from a giant shoe—the hospital dormitory.

HOSPITAL MANAGEMENT

Vol. IX, No. 4
April, 1920

417 S. Dearborn
Street,
Chicago

Published in the Interest of Executives in Every Department of Hospital Work

The Hospital Production Sheet

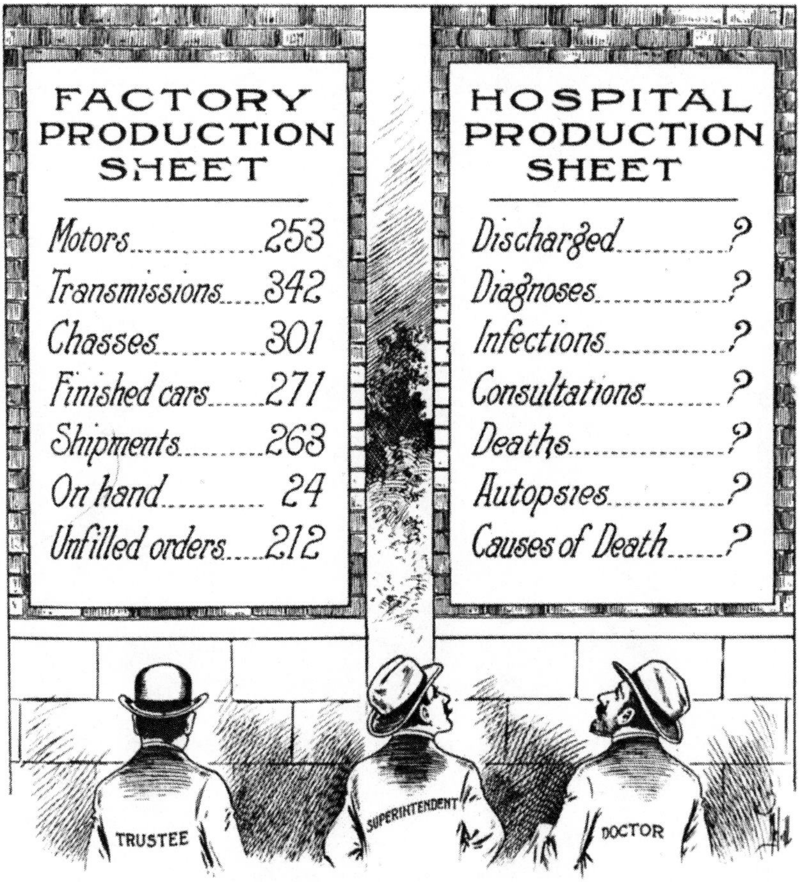

FACTORY
PRODUCTION
SHEET

Motors............253
Transmissions....342
Chasses..........301
Finished cars.....271
Shipments........263
On hand..........24
Unfilled orders...212

HOSPITAL
PRODUCTION
SHEET

Discharged.........?
Diagnoses..........?
Infections.........?
Consultations......?
Deaths.............?
Autopsies..........?
Causes of Death....?

TRUSTEE   SUPERINTENDENT   DOCTOR

FIGURE 1.4.   Cover of *Hospital Management* showing trustee fears about standardized factory-model hospitals.

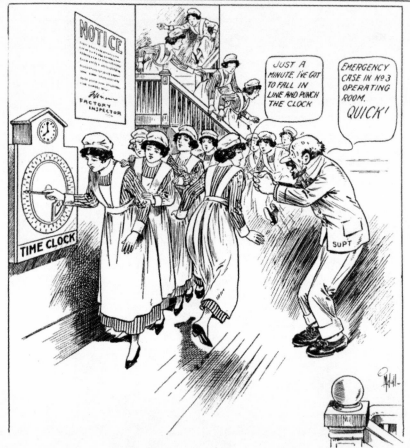

FIGURE 1.5. Cover of *Hospital Management* showing a superintendent pleading with a line of nurses to attend to an emergency case.

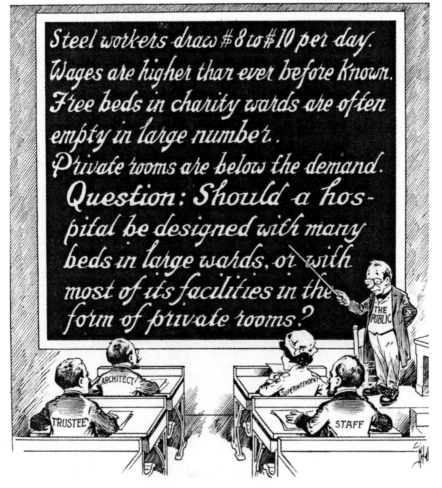

HOSPITAL MANAGEMENT

Vol. VII, No. 3.
October, 1919

417 S. Dearborn
Street,
Chicago

Published in the Interest of Executives in Every Department of Hospital Work

The Class in Hospital Designing

Steel workers draw $8 to $10 per day.
Wages are higher than ever before known.
Free beds in charity wards are often empty in large number.
Private rooms are below the demand.
Question: Should a hospital be designed with many beds in large wards, or with most of its facilities in the form of private rooms?

FIGURE 1.6.   Cover of *Hospital Management* showing the resistance of trustees to the new efficiency model.

November, 1917
Vol. IV, No. 4

HOSPITAL
MANAGEMENT

608 S. Dearborn
Street,
Chicago

Published in the Interest of Executives in Every Department of Hospital Work
Entered as second class matter May 14, 1917, at the post office at Chicago, Ill., under the act of March 3, 1879.

Hospital Service Must Balance Needs of Patient

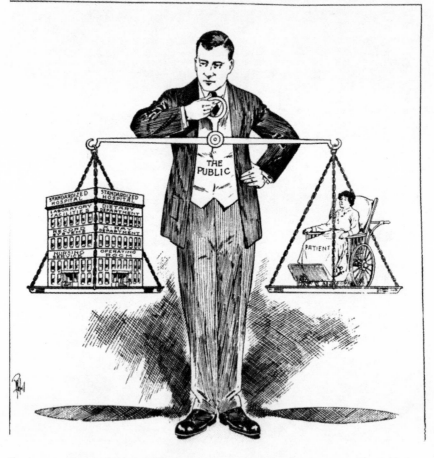

FIGURE 1.7.   Cover of *Hospital Management* showing a man who represents "the public" balancing a scale with the "standardized hospital."

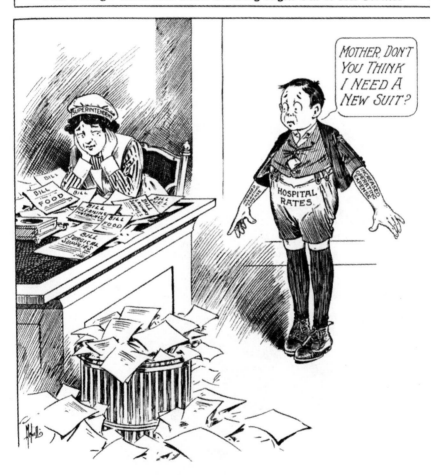

April, 1917
Vol. III, No. 3

HOSPITAL MANAGEMENT

608 S. Dearborn Street, Chicago

Published in the Interest of Executives in Every Department of Hospital Work

This Young Fellow Has Been Growing Right Out of His Clothes

FIGURE 1.8.   Cover of *Hospital Management* showing a female hospital superintendent facing a desk full of bills, while a child labeled "hospital rates" stands by.

Vol. X, No. 2
August, 1920

HOSPITAL MANAGEMENT

417 S. Dearborn
Street,
Chicago

Published in the Interest of Executives in Every Department of Hospital Work

The New Member of the "Team"

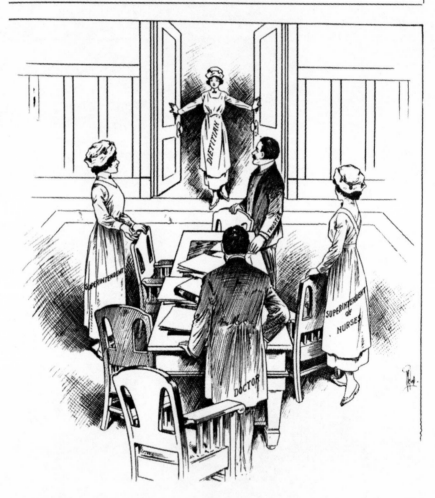

FIGURE 1.9.   Cover of *Hospital Management* showing the new team—trustees, physicians, the superintendent, the superintendent of nurses, and the dietician.

NOTES

1. *Hospital Management* 10, no. 5 (1920). Figures 1.1–1.9 are grouped beginning on p. 30.

2. C. Rosenberg, *The Care of Strangers: The Rise of America's Hospital System* (New York, Basic Books, 1987), 50–51. Rosenberg describes the pious behavior of patients that might inspire trustees to visit them. For example, Rosenberg quotes one trustee at Massachusetts General Hospital as reflecting, "Many a bright version recurs to my imagination of sufferers who, by their truly Christian resignation and fortitude . . . warmly enlisted the sympathy and regard of all who saw them."

3. M. Vogel, *The Invention of the Modern Hospital, Boston 1870–1930* (Chicago: University of Chicago Press, 1980), 13, 27.

4. Rosenberg, *Care of Strangers*, 49.

5. E.g., the creed inscribed over the main entrance of New York's Presbyterian Hospital read, "Presbyterian Hospital—for the poor of New York without regard to Race, Creed, or Color." See D. B. Delavan, *The Early Days of Presbyterian Hospital* (New York: published privately, 1926), 57. Also, Presbyterian Hospital's foundation myth carried by many of the employees argued that founder James Lenox had decided to raise funds for the hospital after one of his African American servants had been denied admission to existing hospitals because of race. See A. Lamb, *The Presbyterian Hospital and the Columbia-Presbyterian Medical Center, 1868–1943* (New York: Columbia University Press, 1955), 11.

6. American Hospital Association.

7. *Hospital Management* 6, no. 4 (1918).

8. *Hospital Management* 3, no. 5 (1917).

9. *Hospital Management* 9, no. 4 (1920).

10. *Hospital Management* 7, no. 3 (1919).

11. D. Rosner, *A Once Charitable Enterprise* (Cambridge: Cambridge University Press, 1982), 22.

12. *Hospital Management* 4, no. 4 (1917).

13. *Hospital Management* 3, no. 3 (1917).

14. D. Rosner, "Doing Well or Doing Good: The Ambivalent Focus of Hospital Administration," in *The American General Hospital*, ed. D. Long and J. Golden (Ithaca, N.Y.: Cornell University Press, 1989), 157–69.

15. May Ayres Burgess as quoted in M. Davis, *Hospital Administration* (New York, 1929), 29.

16. As quoted in Davis, *Hospital Administration*, 30.

17. Rosner, "Doing Well or Doing Good."

18. D. Rosner, "Heterogeneity and Uniformity," in *In Sickness and in Health*, ed. J. D. Seay and B. C. Vladeck (New York: McGraw-Hill, 1988), 87–125, at 101.

19. Richard Shryock, *The Development of Modern Medicine* (Madison: University of Wisconsin Press, 1979), 143.

20. *Hospital Management* 3, no. 5 (1917).

21. *Hospital Management* 10, no. 2 (1920).

22. Allen R. Myerson, "When Healing Collides with the Drive for Profits," *New York Times*, July 27, 1997, section 1, p. 14.

23. Rosner, *Once Charitable Enterprise*, 187–91.

24. Annette Fuentes and Rosemary Metzler Lavan, "No Health, No Wealth," *The Nation,* December 18, 2000, 11. They state: "Since 1980, when the election of Ronald Reagan ushered in an era of free-market, privatized economics, more than 400 hospitals and more than a dozen health plans have converted to for-profit status."

25. *New York Times,* April 11, 1997.

26. *New York Times,* April 11, 1997.

27. *New York Times,* July 27, 1997.

2

THE LEGAL RESPONSIBILITIES OF VOLUNTARY HOSPITAL TRUSTEES

J. David Seay

Managers of hospitals and other nonprofit organizations often hear such anecdotes as "I have trouble recruiting some of the best potential trustees because they are afraid of the liability," or "The first question my new trustee prospects ask is 'Do you carry directors and officers liability insurance?'" Whether these prospective trustees are feigning the fear of personal liability as an excuse to say no may never be known. But it is a good bet that at least some of them are truly worried that serving as a trustee will expose them to the potential risk of personal liability. The phenomenon has found its way into the popular press, as well.[1] This is especially so in the case of the large and complex organization known as the modern hospital, where the potential of medical malpractice and personnel injury hangs in the air. How real are those fears and how justified are those who decline to serve their communities in these important positions?

This chapter explores the legal framework for the responsibilities of the voluntary hospital trustee, and hence it can be instructive as to the potentiality of personal risk and liability. The terms "trustee" and "director" are both used herein, and they are for all intents and purposes interchangeable, notwithstanding their historical differences. This chapter is written upon the premise that better informed and educated trustees will result in better governance and better hospitals, and will decrease the likelihood of personal liability arising from hospital trusteeship.

Why are the legal duties and responsibilities of hospital trusteeship important? First of all, these legal rules or boundaries form the basis upon which legal liability may be based. The legal duties and responsibilities are, simply put, the standards by which a trustee's behavior may be judged. They therefore can provide some important guidance on what role a trustee plays relative to management and others involved with the hospital, including patients, employees, competitors, and others within the community more broadly.

The legal duties and responsibilities of hospital trustees are also important to many individuals in the community or communities served by the hospital in that they—and hospital trusteeship itself—can provide them with a vehicle through which they can discharge their sense of social and community responsibility. Voluntary service to all types of nonprofit, charitable organizations can provide an outlet for this uniquely American impulse to serve and to "give back" something to the communities in which individuals have grown and prospered. The motivations for hospital trusteeship are varied, of course, but altruism remains prominent among them.

These standards can also offer a framework for evaluating the success or failure of trustee actions, either individually or collectively, though many hospitals and trustees shy away from an active and effective use of the standards for this purpose. However, if done carefully and appropriately, the legal duties and responsibilities of hospital trusteeship can be a highly effective tool in reviewing and evaluating governance performance.[2] In a very real sense, then, this chapter is designed as an introductory or primer course in hospital trusteeship so that the basics of hospital trustee duty, responsibility, and liability can be better understood.

The law pertaining to the legal responsibilities of hospital trustees comes from numerous sources. Principal among those sources are statutory laws and implementing regulations, at both the state and federal levels, such as those enforced by state departments of health and the U.S. Department of Health and Human Services. There is also case law or common law history and precedent, used both by judges deciding certain types of suits brought against charitable organizations and their trustees, and by state attorneys general exercising their oversight responsibility of trusts and charitable entities in their respective states. And there are also administrative laws, such as those enforced by such agencies as the Internal Revenue Service, which pertain to the nonprofit sector and are a significant source of the law in this area. This chapter draws from these sources of law in examining the duties and responsibilities of hospital trustees.[3]

The Basics of Trusteeship

So just what are the "basics" of hospital trusteeship and trustee liability? Trusteeship involves duties and responsibilities, the breach of which can result in liability. However, the potential for individual trustee liability and the potential for institutional liability must not be confused. Organizations such as hospitals are sued all the time for a whole manner of alleged wrongs, including employment issues such as alleged sexual harassment, contract disputes, medical malpractice, and other personal injuries. In those "third-party" suits, the entity most often sued is the hospital entity or corporation itself, and not the board, either collectively or individually. And hospitals carry all kinds of liability insurance to cover for any successful suits in these areas.

With some exceptions, trustees are rarely, if ever, sued in such matters. As will be made clear later in this chapter, one reason for this is that the classes of persons permitted "standing" by the law to sue directors and officers of corporations are indeed limited. And further, as shall be described, the standards of behavior for directors and officers are such that injury or other wrongful acts can in fact occur in the absence of culpability ascribed to the directors and officers, as long as they had properly discharged their duties and responsibilities to the corporation and had acted in good faith. However, there remain certain types of lawsuits that can properly name trustees as defendants, and this section will examine what they are, what the standards of behavior are, and how a trustee can best minimize his or her own exposure to personal liability.

Basically, three "rules of thumb" are important for trustees to follow: (1) Be there; that is, show up at board and committee meetings and actively participate in board deliberations. (2) Ask questions. This is one of the most fundamental tasks a trustee should accomplish. Because trustees are not involved—and should not be involved—in the management and day-to-day operations of the hospital, they cannot exert many of the types of controls with which they may be familiar. Asking questions and inquiring of management into the meaning of information provided to them and into the nature of proposed initiatives often forms the basis of good trustee behavior, and can protect the trustee in that such behavior can discharge the trustee's duty and responsibility. And (3) avoid conflicts of interest above all else: Disclose and abstain. Where a conflict of interest, a potential conflict of interest, or even the appearance of a conflict of interest may arise in the course of serving on a hospital board, at a minimum the trustee must disclose his or her interest—real, potential, or apparent—and abstain from voting on that matter. In some states stricter rules apply, but in New York and some other jurisdictions, disclosure and abstention are sufficient to immunize a trustee from liability in such instances.

"How Do You Sue Me? Let Me Count the Ways"

So, just why *do* trustees get sued? There are three primary types of lawsuits against the directors and officers of hospitals and other types of nonprofit, charitable organizations. (1) Lawsuits alleging a breach of one or more of the various duties and responsibilities of trusteeship—the principal focus of this chapter—are one type of action that can be taken against trustees. Although the class of individuals who can bring these types of suits is small, the risk is real and an understanding of the duties and standards of behavior is important to properly discharging trustee duties and avoiding personal liability. (2) Third-party lawsuits, which were referred to above, are suits brought by individuals or entities outside the hospital alleging some wrongdoing or injury. "Slip-and-fall" cases are examples, as are wrongful discharges from employment and the like. Most often, it is the institution itself that is named as the party defendant to these cases, and not the individual trustee or trustees. However, because responsibility for the activity of the medical staff ultimately rests with the board of trustees, the trustees are often made party to malpractice suits, although the hospital most often defends against these actions and indemnifies and holds trustees harmless from such suits, so long as the trustees were acting in good faith in the discharge of their individual and collective duties and responsibilities as trustees in the selection and monitoring of the qualifications and behavior of the medical staff. (3) The third type of lawsuit involves statutory violations or breaches of the common law governing charitable organizations. These types of suits are brought by the attorney general of the state having jurisdiction over the hospital and who have broad powers in overseeing such charities and activities.

This area of the law is analogous to tort law that asserts, in essence, where the law imposes a duty, such as a duty to act in a certain way, there then arises the potential for a breach of that duty.[4] If a breach of the duty occurs, and if there is resultant harm or injury, and if it can be shown that the harm or injury was directly caused by the breach, then liability can be found. In the hospital trusteeship context, by agreeing to become a hospital trustee, one by implication agrees to be held to certain standards of care, for the breach of which one can be held liable if harm results. In many cases of director and officer liability, the alleged harm is not to third parties but rather to the institution or hospital itself. In such suits, the hospital itself is alleged to have been harmed by the director or officer failing to live up to the legally imposed standards of behavior.

"Standing" is the legal term relating to who can or is in a position to sue another party. Fortunately, under our system of laws, not just anyone can sue anyone else whenever they feel like it, contrary to popular belief. For example, both parties to a contract have equal standing to sue each other over an alleged breach. An unrelated third party lacks a relationship to the agreement and thus is not accorded standing to sue. And although there may be many persons with a desire to sue a hospital, those with standing to sue directors and officers of the hospital are usually few and far between.

The pool of potential plaintiffs in director and officer litigation traditionally has been limited to the following four classes.[5] (1) First "members" of a corporation may sue its directors and officers. Many charitable corporations historically were organized as membership corporations, often with several classes of individuals designated among various classes of members of the corporation. Also called "voting members," these individuals are analogous to shareholders in the for-profit corporation, and their rights are generally limited to electing the directors of the hospital or other such membership corporation. Some states, like New York, for years required all charitable corporations to be formed as membership corporations. New York amended its law some years ago to allow charitable corporations to be formed as "corporations without members," in which the boards of directors are essentially self-perpetuating in that they elect their own successor trustees.[6] (2) The second class of individuals with standing to sue are other trustees and officers of the same organization. (3) The third are the attorneys general of the states in which nonprofits are incorporated. They have been granted standing under the common law, and in some instances, statutes to, in effect, sue as proxies on behalf of the "beneficiaries" of the hospital—the people of the community or communities served by the institution. (4) The fourth category of persons sometimes given standing to sue includes individuals with particular or unusually close relationships with the organization, such as a founder or, in some rare instances, a major benefactor.

That is it. Those, with some rare exceptions, are the categories of people who can sue individuals for failing to do their jobs appropriately as directors and officers. Some of the exceptions include former patients of a hospital—as seen in the *Sibley Hospital* case[7]—who charged the board with improper inside dealing at the expense of the hospital, which, in turn, had to raise its rates to patients. Another exception was granted to college students—as seen with the *Wilson College* case[8]—where the school's board of trustees was moving to close the school for financial reasons after having made no attempts to solve its fiscal problems. In both cases, the courts reacted to clear cases of especially egregious behavior. Granting standing to the particular classes of individuals seeking to sue was the only way serious wrongs could be righted. There have been very few such instances since these cases, making it clear both that expanding standing to sue is the exception rather than the rule, and that, nonetheless, it can be done where the trustees' actions are wrong and reckless, where irreparable harm will result, and where there is no other recourse available. In most states, the more restrictive standard of who can sue directors and officers still stands.

With respect to hospital trustees, there is another "exception" in medical malpractice suits. Because the ultimate responsibility for patient care—and the organized medical staff—lies with the board and is considered a board responsibility, in many cases and in some jurisdictions malpractice suits brought against the hospital may also include the trustees as parties defendant. Because this type of responsibility falls within the usual duties of trustees, such suits are routinely covered by the hospital's own liability insurance policies and indemnification procedures.

TRUSTEESHIP IS A LOT LIKE MARRIAGE

When the legal duties of trustees are examined, it looks a lot like a marriage. The basic legal duties include the duties of care, loyalty, and obedience—similar to the marital vows to love, honor, and obey. And in today's rapidly changing, evolving, and complex health care marketplace—including hospitals' involvement in myriad new corporate arrangements and relationships—the duties of a trustee become heightened because it is just simply a lot easier to miss something important or be asleep at the switch when major decisions are made. Trustees may therefore be liable for their inaction as much as their actions.[9]

This section examines the three duties of care, obedience, and loyalty, in that order, and attempts to both explain them in everyday terms while at the same time providing some practical tips toward compliance. These duties form the backbone of the legal basis for hospital trustees' responsibilities.

The Duty of Care

The duty of care, derived from common-law case decisions, sets forth the legal minimum behavior for a trustee or director to follow to fully discharge his or her responsibilities as a fiduciary. A fiduciary is someone charged with acting on behalf of another or an institution. The duty or "standard of care" is defined as that behavior or action that an ordinarily prudent person would ordinarily undertake in similar circumstances.

What that means in practical terms is that the trustee must at all times act with informed and independent judgment in his or her capacity as a trustee of the hospital. Informed means that trustees have an affirmative duty to review information provided to them by the management of the hospital and to request additional information and data that they determine may be helpful in informing their decisions. There are growing burdens in this area, as reflected by some recent cases requiring the creation and use of information and compliance systems within the institution to inform management and the governing board.[10] Another practical requirement is active attendance at, and participation in, board and committee meetings. One cannot discharge one's legal duties of trusteeship in absentia, and some states prohibit trustees from voting by proxy. Thus, trustees can be liable for bad decisions in which they did not even participate. These last two practical requirements are reflective of what was meant earlier in the general rule of thumb to "be there and ask questions."

The duty of care also requires a trustee's behavior or actions to be made in good faith. By that it is meant that the trustee must at all times act openly, with pure intent, and with the institution's best interests in mind. Fair and arm's-length dealing with the hospital and related entities is required of all trustees. An otherwise legitimate vote made by a trustee, for example, may violate the duty of care, as well as one or more of the other duties, if that decision also enriches or otherwise benefits the trustee in a secret or undisclosed manner. This can be true even if the hospital is not materially harmed by such action. The trustee must undertake due care in the best interests of the hospital only.[11]

The law also extends a broad degree of protection to trustees acting in good faith. A legal doctrine called the "business judgment rule" has been created by common-law court decisions, arising largely out of cases dealing with business corporations. This rule, in essence, says that courts will not entertain lawsuits against directors and officers, or otherwise look over the shoulder of and second guess the business judgments of such directors and officers, as long as they were acting in good faith, unless there is some egregious or otherwise compelling reason to do so.[12] Wide latitude is thus given to the actions and decisions of directors and officers of hospitals, and other corporations, in areas where the courts do not presuppose as much as or more knowledge than those directors and officers engaged in a particular business or activity. The business judgment rule can provide great solace to nervous directors and officers of hospitals, fearing that lawsuits may meet many of their more controversial and difficult decisions. This may be particularly true in decisions to downsize, merge, or otherwise consolidate or affiliate with other institutions, or to sell out to or convert to for-profit status, in jurisdictions where that is allowed. State attorneys general, however, may have jurisdiction over some of those examples, and many around the country have become active in policing some of them, especially conversions and sales to proprietary firms. Even in those cases, if litigation is pursued by the attorney general, the business judgment rule may be a helpful defense that can be used by the corporation and directors and officers so challenged.

The Duty of Obedience

The duty of obedience finds its derivation in the law of trusts, wherein trustees are bound by the law to be obedient to the stated intentions of the testator—or creator of the trust—and carry out the purposes of the trust exactly as intended.[13] In this sense, then, and in the context of hospital trusteeship, "mission matters," a topic visited earlier by this author and others.[14] Most hospitals, however, have no one creator or benefactor from whom to draw mission, and in fact, the hospital may have had hundreds of benefactors over the years as well as a mission altered by the dictates of time and changing demographics of the communities served by the hospital, among other intervening factors. Therefore a hospital trustee's responsibility here is really a double duty. It includes both interpreting and redefining mission in evolving and changing circumstances and being obedient to that mission. A hospital without a mission statement, or an outmoded or overly general one that offers scant guidance, may become seriously adrift in the roiling seas of contemporary health care. Trustees are, in essence, the conscience of the hospital for it is incumbent upon them to both articulate and follow mission.

To qualify as tax exempt, the Internal Revenue Code requires a hospital or other charity to be both organized and operated as a public charity and community-benefit organization.[15] The first part, the "organizational test," is met by the hospital being incorporated as a not-for-profit corporation under the relevant state law, among other things, and the second part, the "operational test," is satisfied only if the hospital is actually run as a charitable or community-benefit institution.[16] Because nonexempt hospitals may also pursue a mission of, for instance, simply "providing hospital services," a voluntary, tax-exempt hospital must do something more—community benefit—to meet the operational test under the law.[17] This is where mission, and a strict adherence to it, are important and where the trustees' duty of obedience can be exercised.

The Duty of Loyalty

The duty of loyalty requires that a trustee be loyal to the hospital and to the hospital alone at all times he or she is acting in the capacity as trustee.[18] A hospital trustee frequently may wear several hats. She may wear the hat of a vendor to the hospital, such as a supply or equipment company owner or executive, or the hat of a banker with whom the hospital has financial relationships, or the hat of an attorney or accountant whose firm represents the hospital. The trustee may wear the hat of a real estate investor or broker who may stand to benefit from a relationship with the hospital. Especially in smaller communities where the potential pool of hospital trustees is limited, there may be many hats involved. However, the duty of loyalty is quite simple. When it comes to hospital trusteeship, you may wear but one hat at a time. When you are in the hospital boardroom or anywhere acting on behalf of the hospital as a trustee, that must be the trustee hat.

The duty of loyalty, then, is the duty that prohibits conflicts of interests. More accurately, this means (in most jurisdictions) avoiding acting on a conflict of interest, as opposed to the mere existence or appearance of a conflict. In many states, such as New York, the presence of a conflict of interest alone is not illegal. It is the failure to disclose one's interest, and acting upon or acquiescing in an action on it, that is considered a violation of the duty of loyalty. This refers back to the general rule of thumb mentioned at the outset, to "disclose and abstain." There is a growing trend, however, to avoid even the appearance of, or a potential, conflict of interest on nonprofit boards even when the law may allow them. Therefore, many boards are discontinuing the practice of having their outside counsel, banker, or anyone else with an interest serve on the governing board. There are myriad ways to tap into the resources and talent of such individuals, such as advisory boards, president's councils, work groups, committees, and the like, without having them serve as trustees.

Breaches of the duty of loyalty can also occur in instances where no boardroom vote is even taken. For example, the appropriation of a business opportunity from the hospital, by virtue (surely that is not the best word choice) of knowledge gained by being a trustee of the hospital can be just as violative of the duty as an outright vote to give hospital business to the bank where you are an officer. Also, you can violate the duty of loyalty by misusing your position as a director or officer of the hospital by using your position to influence a particular decision that may turn out to benefit you or an organization—even another charity—with which you are affiliated.

The duty of loyalty demands a trustee's undivided allegiance to the hospital, and courts have placed a stricter scrutiny on nonprofit trustees in this area. In general, no trustee should receive any pecuniary gain from board service other than reimbursement of legitimate expenses or directors fees. Historically, nonprofit trustees have not been compensated for their service as trustees, with an exception being trustees of private foundations. In fact, at least one state prohibits it entirely,[19] and some states impose limits in certain areas.[20] In most cases, however, it is legal to compensate trustees, and a few hospitals and systems have begun to do so, and some commentators think it is a good idea.[21]

Some jurisdictions have also adopted certain statutory provisions prohibiting or regulating certain specific aspects related to the duty of loyalty. For example, some states statutorily prohibit conflicts of interest, and others forbid such things as loans to officers and directors.[22]

In a nutshell, the best way to assure compliance with the duty of loyalty is to know the specifics of a particular state's laws governing not-for-profit corporations, and to disclose and abstain from voting in instances in which one has an interest.

PROTECTIONS FOR TRUSTEES

The protections of the business judgment rule have already been discussed. What happens, though, when despite the best of intentions and the business judgment rule, violations of the duties of a trustee might have occurred? And, are there things that can be done to lessen the chance of such occurrences? Are there any other forms of protection to assuage the fear of the apprehensive trustee?

There are several additional types of protection of which trustees and institutions can avail themselves, including insurance, indemnification, and certain "risk management-like" techniques. Each can help to ease the minds of hospital trustees, though each has its limits.

Insurance for Directors and Officers

Liability insurance coverage for directors and officers—"D&O coverage"—is a type of insurance that covers both judgments obtained against a trustee or trustees for wrongs they may have committed against the hospital, and the costs of defending such suits, up to certain specified limits contained in the individual policies. There is both good and bad news in the D&O coverage area. The good news is that, overall, the premiums for such coverage have been decreasing in recent years from the highs of a few years ago, although that will vary from industry to industry, hospital to hospital, and, like most insurance, can be experience-rated—which means much higher premiums for hospitals that have had significant adverse D&O claims experience. The bad news is that there have been recent trends to limit coverage or protection under such policies. It is very important to read these policies carefully to ascertain just what is covered and what is not.

Most good D&O policies cover claims arising from wrongful acts or omissions, or other breaches of duty by trustees. However, there are often a number of exclusions. Common examples of such exclusions include claims for bodily injury or property damage. Damages of this type should be insured separately, most often under a general or umbrella liability policy. Self-dealing by or among trustees is also frequently excluded from many D&O policies. This is a significant exclusion, given the new intermediate sanction regulations recently promulgated by the Internal Revenue Service pertaining to 501(c)(3) and (4) organizations.[23] Some policies have been specifically designed, at the insistence of nonprofit umbrella groups, to include intermediate sanction-type wrongs in D&O policies, as long as trustees are acting in good faith, and any excise taxes or fines levied are the result of mistake or unintentional error on the part of the trustee or trustees.[24]

Another common exclusion of D&O policies is for claims seeking other than monetary damages. Nonmonetary damage claims include claims for specific performance of contracts, that is, claims seeking to compel compliance with an existing contractual obligation as opposed to seeking to void the contract and seek liquidated damages. Temporary restraining orders or other types of injunctive relief, where the court's help is sought to either make someone or some entity do or stop doing a particular thing, are other examples, as are claims seeking to reinstate an employee alleging wrongful discharge from employment.

And, the last examples of common exclusions are claims wherein the willful violation of a statute committed by or with the knowledge or consent of a trustee has occurred. Few D&O policies will cover such behavior.

The practical result of all of these exclusions is that coverage is then generally limited to money damage claims against trustees for injuring the corporation itself in situations other than self-dealing (e.g., mismanagement of funds or improper use of restricted funds). Despite the coverage limitations, for a number of reasons it still may be a wise decision for a hospital to purchase good D&O liability insurance coverage.

One very good reason to do so is to avail the trustee and the hospital of the legal defense cost coverage offered by most D&O policies, because the cost of defending such litigation can be substantial—even if the trustees and the hospital ultimately prevail in the litigation. But even here, there are contract limitations in coverage. For example, most policies cap or otherwise limit the total amount of such defense coverage, and deductibles are frequently used to, in effect, share the costs. Additionally, policy language will often limit the policyholder's ability to unilaterally select the attorneys who will represent them. Some policies require that the insurer select defense counsel, while others merely give them a sign-off or veto power over counsel selected by the policyholder.

Legal costs are mostly covered for trustees arising from claims made against them for which they are not indemnified by the hospital. Under those types of policies, if the hospital pays, then the policy does not. Some policies pay claims directly, while others reimburse the trustee or hospital for claims paid by them. Some policies cover only the trustees or directors, and not the institution itself, so policies should be read carefully to see if "entity coverage" is included or excluded.

Care must also be taken in determining whether the coverage is for "claims-made" or "occurrence-made" coverage. In "claims-made" policies, the carrier must be notified of any claim made during the period the policy is or was in effect, and the coverage will extend to the date the claim was made only in such instances. In the more common or traditional "occurrence-made" policies, the coverage applies for occurrences of covered events during the effective date of the policy, even though the claim may be asserted or filed after the policy has terminated. With respect to all of the coverage and exclusions herein discussed, it is important that all such policies be periodically reviewed as insurance trends and legal mandates change. And it is also important to periodically review the market for new products and policies coming onto the market.

Indemnification of Directors and Officers

Some hospitals and other nonprofit, charitable organizations are allowed to indemnify their directors and officers. Indemnification simply means that the hospital will pay claims and costs of defense for their directors and officers when they are sued in that capacity. Often these payments are, like D&O coverage, limited to certain situations in which willful wrongdoing or gross negligence is absent. Frequently, state statutes governing not-for-profit corporations will dictate exactly what types of actions or omissions can be covered by indemnification. Also, it is common for statutes to allow hospitals to indemnify, but not without some formalities. These types of statutes are merely permissive in nature. For example, a statute may allow indemnification but require that the organization's own governing documents, such as the by-laws, be amended to effectuate such coverage.[25]

Clearly, both D&O insurance and indemnification can be beneficial to both the directors and officers of a hospital, as well as the hospital itself. Many hospitals use both to effectuate optimal coverage. Care should be taken, though, to assure that both types of policies dovetail and are consistent and do not conflict with or duplicate each other.

Risk Management Techniques

Risk management, in its simplest description, is the prevention of losses before they occur. In that sense, it is the most efficient of the protections available to hospital trustees. Just as risk management techniques can work to prevent slips and falls on just-mopped hospital corridors by the use of signage and warnings, so also can analogous techniques assist inside the hospital's boardroom. The best way to achieve risk management in the governance context is through education and information. A better informed and educated trustee—barring intentional wrongdoing—is going to be far less likely to run afoul of the governance duties and responsibilities that are the subject of this chapter.

Trustee education is often difficult to achieve. Trustees are busy and important people whose time and schedules are short and crowded. Efforts to pursue effective hospital trustee continuing education through external or third-party organizations outside the hospital have met with mixed success, and hospitals' own trustee education goals have also been a challenge in many instances. One approach, in addition to continuing education programs, is to build some information and trustee education into the hospital's trustee selection and recruitment process. Another is to add a board and trustee evaluation component into the annual or biannual governance calendar. Much information can be contained in both types of activity that can further the goals of trustee education, and in turn, governance risk management.

As far as good programs and high-quality educational materials for hospital trustees are concerned, several national and local resources exist. BoardSource, formerly the National Center for Nonprofit Boards, publishes a wide array of governance-related materials for all nonprofits, as do the Nonprofit Risk Management Center and the Peter F. Drucker Foundation for Nonprofit Management,[26] which has produced some excellent board self-assessment tools. High-quality programs and published materials designed exclusively for hospital trustees are available from the national organization Volunteer Trustees of Not-for-Profit Hospitals,[27] which has also done some exceptional work relating to the sale and conversion of not-for-profit hospitals to for-profits.

Other organizations also provide related materials and programs, including statewide organizations such as Healthcare Trustees of New York State, and metropolitan ones such as the Nonprofit Coordinating Committee of New York and the United Hospital Fund. Many other states and localities have similar organizations. Also at the national level, the Support Centers of America, Foundation Center, and Council on Foundations have produced information and programs helpful to nonprofit trustees.

A few specific publications are worthy of mention here as very good primary source documents for hospital trustees. They include the already mentioned Kurtz book,[28] a guidebook for nonprofit directors by the American Bar Association,[29] and a useful booklet on risk management by a major insurer.[30]

TRENDS TO KEEP AN EYE ON

There are a few emerging trends in trustee liability worthy of scrutiny. Among them are a couple of seemingly contradictory trends. One is to liberalize or loosen the standards of care for nonprofit trustees,[31] in an effort to remove a perceived "chilling effect" on trusteeship arising from the fear of personal liability. The notion is that if the potential for trustee liability were lessened, more people would be willing to serve in that capacity.

On the other hand is the trend demanding greater accountability from nonprofit organizations arising from high-profile cases of board impropriety, such as the Boston University and Adelphi University cases, as well as the United

Way of America and the Bishop Estate foundation in Hawaii, among others, and from the feeling that some hospitals and other nonprofits are not doing their fair share of "charity" when it is defined as poverty-reducing activities.[32] And it is not insignificant that many local tax assessors and politicians see gold in revoking tax exemptions from hospitals at a time when revenues from other sources are shrinking and the demand for public services is increasing. Court decisions, administrative rule making, new and proposed legislation at both the state and federal levels, and public opinion samples have all confirmed an increasing demand for more disclosure and accountability among hospitals and other nonprofit organizations.

Other trends to keep an eye on include an increasing number of lawsuits brought against hospitals for alleged wrongful terminations of employment. This is a trend in almost all sectors, but for hospital trustees it can be particularly active and thorny because of the board's duty to actively oversee the medical staff and its various processes, including terminations and other disciplinary actions. There are also increasing numbers of sexual harassment law suits, some of which may involve suits against directors and officers, depending on the circumstances and category of employee.

Another trend, also involving physicians, but involving increasing numbers of other health care professionals within the ambit of hospitals, systems, and managed care organizations as well, is toward more allegations of wrongdoing in relation to the credentialing of health care professionals. As the number of these suits increase, the likelihood of directors and officers suits also increases, especially with respect to physician credentialing decisions—again because of the board's role in ultimately assuring the quality and competence of the hospital's medical staff.

Further, as alluded to above, the trend toward greater scrutiny of all areas relating to tax-exempt status will continue.[33] Intermediate sanction regulations, referred to above, will not make these problems go away. In addition to private inurnment problems (where individuals improperly benefit at the expense of the hospital)—only some of which will be covered by the new regulations—there are private benefit issues (where the class of persons served by the corporation is too small), and lingering concerns over whether the hospital provides enough community benefit and how that is defined. The new disclosure requirement regulations,[34] which facilitate easier access to hospitals' Internal Revenue Service Form 990,[35] which includes salary information for top employees, will likely fuel more allegations of excessive executive and physician compensation, while at the same time letting more sunshine in on hospital financial and programmatic operations. And hospitals, like other nonprofits, will continue periodically to be criticized by politicians and others for lobbying and political activities, which some believe to be inappropriate activities for organizations that are public charities, and subsidized, some would argue, by the effect of tax-exempt status.

I conclude with the observation that like marriage, trusteeship can be a very rich and rewarding experience, but not one without its own duties and responsibilities. The duties to love, honor, and obey in marriage—and to live up to the legal duties of care, loyalty, and obedience to a hospital or other public charity—do have certain analogies and similarities. Hospital trusteeship can be both a serious responsibility, on the one hand, and on the other a source of public service, volunteerism, charity, and gratification. Potential trustees need not be scared away from trusteeship by misconceptions and misinformation about the risk of personal liability.

I began, and now end, with the premise that a better informed trustee can lead to better governance, decreased risks of personal liability, and better health care through a better run hospital or health care system. The simple rule of thumb recited at the outset—to "be there, ask questions, and avoid conflicts"—can go a long way in helping a hospital trustee to better discharge his or her legal responsibilities. This, plus keeping an eye on the important trends that will be making an impact on hospital governance and the decisions hospital trustees must make on behalf of their institutions, will promote better trustee education and better governed hospitals.

NOTES

1. "Board Members Draw Fire and Some Think Twice about Serving," *Wall Street Journal*, February 5, 1986, 1.

2. Dennis D. Pointer and James E. Orlikoff, *Board Work: Governing Health Care Organizations* (San Francisco: Jossey-Bass, 1999); John Carver, *Boards That Make a Difference* (San Francisco: Jossey-Bass, 1990).

3. A number of overview documents and resources are available for supplemental reading, including an excellent book devoted to trustee liability, which was instructive to this author in the preparation of this chapter. See Daniel L. Kurtz, *Board Liability: A Guide for Nonprofit Directors* (Mount Kisco, N.Y.: Moyer Bell Ltd., 1988).

4. Marion Fremont-Smith, "Enforceability and Sanctions," presentation at a conference, Governance of Nonprofit Organizations: Standards and Enforcement, New York University School of Law, National Center on Philanthropy and the Law, New York, October 30–31, 1997.

5. Kurtz, *Board Liability*, 92.

6. N.Y. Not-for-Profit Corp. L. (N.Y. N-PCL), Sec. 601.

7. *Stern v. Lucy Webb Hayes National Training School*, 367 F. Supp. 536 (D.D.C. 1973), 381 F. Supp.10003 (D.D.C. 1974), commonly referred to as the *Sibley Hospital* case; Kurtz, *Board Liability*, 93.

8. *Zehner v. Alexander*, No. 56, 1979, slip op. (Comm. Plea, 39th Dist. Pa., 1979), commonly referred to as the *Wilson College* case.

9. Evelyn Brody, "The Limits of Charity Fiduciary Law," *Maryland Law Review* 57 (1998): 1400.

10. In Re Caremark International, Inc. Derivative Litigation, 698 A.2d 959 (1997).

11. Kurtz, *Board Liability*, 22–48.

12. Kurtz, *Board Liability*, 49–59.

13. Kurtz, *Board Liability*, 84–90.

14. J. David Seay and Bruce C. Vladeck, "Mission Matters" in *In Sickness and in Health: The Mission of Voluntary Health Care Institutions*, ed. Seay and Vladeck (New York: McGraw-Hill, 1988), 1.

15. Internal Revenue Code, Sec. 501(c)(3).

16. "Charity," in its legal definition within the hospital context, does not mean the relief of poverty, per se, but rather is defined by the historical concept of "other purposes beneficial to the community"; hence the term "community benefit."

17. J. David Seay, "Tax Exemption for Hospitals: Towards an Understanding of Community Benefit," *Health Matrix* 2, no 35 (1992): 45–48; and J. David Seay and Robert M. Sigmond, "Community Benefit Standards for Hospitals: Perceptions and Performance," *Frontiers of Health Services Management* 5, no. 3 (spring 1989): 3–39.

18. Kurtz, *Board Liability*, 59–84.

19. Ohio Rev. Code Sec. 1713.30.

20. N.Y. Ment. Hyg. L. Sec. 75.15; 27 NYCRR 75.

21. Ira Millstein, "Lesson for For-Profit Governance: Responsibilities in the Hospital Boardroom," presentation at United Hospital Fund of New York's Trustee Leadership Briefing Series, New York, February 19, 1998.

22. N.Y. N-PCL, Sec. 716.

23. Taxpayer Bill of Rights 2 (P.L. 104–168, 1996); Internal Revenue Code, 26 U.S.C. 4958, REG-246256–96 (1998).

24. E.g., the Nonprofit Coordinating Committee of New York has crafted a D&O coverage policy with nonprofits in mind, and includes intermediate sanction coverage, as well as a number of technical improvements that are beneficial to nonprofit organizations. The group has also negotiated a very reasonable premium level for these policies.

25. N.Y. N-PCL, Sec. 721 et seq.

26. BoardSource, 1828 L Street, N.W., Washington, D.C. 20036; Nonprofit Risk Management Center, 1001 Connecticut Avenue, N.W., Suite 900, Washington, D.C. 20036; Peter F. Drucker Foundation for Nonprofit Management, 320 Park Avenue, New York, N.Y. 10022.

27. Volunteer Trustees of Not-for-Profit Hospitals, 818 18th Street, N.W., Suite 900, Washington, D.C. 20006.

28. Kurtz, *Board Liability*.

29. George W. Overton, ed., *Guidebook for Directors of Nonprofit Corporations, Section on Business Law, Nonprofit Corporations Committee* (Chicago: American Bar Association, 1993).

30. Dan A. Bailey, *Directors & Officers Liability: Loss Prevention for Nonprofit Organizations* (Warren, N.J.: Chubb & Son, Inc., 1989).

31. See generally the Uniform Management of Institutional Funds Act, the "prudent investor rule," and proposed legislation to lower the standard of care for all nonprofit, charitable trustees.

32. Letter of Agreement between the Commonwealth of Massachusetts, Office of the Attorney General and Dr. G. B. Metcalf, Chairman and on behalf of Trustees of Boston University (November 16, 1993). *Committee to Save Adelphi, et al. v. Diamandopoulos, et al., Board of Regents of the State of New York* (February 5, 1997). *U.S. v. Aramony, et al.*, 88F3d. 1369 (1996), and related cases. "Trustees Ousted in Hawaii," *Chronicle of Philanthropy* 11, no. 15 (1999).

33. John D. Colombo and Mark A. Hall, *The Charitable Tax Exemption* (Boulder, Colo.: Westview Press, 1995).

34. Internal Revenue Code Sec. 6104(e)91)(A)(i).

35. Internal Revenue Service Form 990, Return of Organization Exempt from Income Tax, Office of Management and Budget No. 1545–0047.

3

HOSPITAL TRUSTEESHIP IN AN ERA OF INSTITUTIONAL TRANSITION

What Can We Learn from Governance Research?

Jeffrey A. Alexander

Governing American hospitals and their related organizational forms is arguably one of the most complex and challenging activities in modern organizational life. These challenges stem from multiple factors, such as the mutually dependent (and changing) relationship between the hospital and its medical staff, the advances and rapid obsolescence of medical technology, the mix of professional and technical personnel necessary to deliver high-quality medical care, and, perhaps most important, the fundamental changes in the role and mission of hospitals as they confront an increasingly competitive marketplace.

Few would dispute the claim that hospitals are facing profound changes, as the economic and social expectations in place in the health care sector have been turned on their heads by funding cuts, managed care, new regulations, vertical integration, and the rise of community-based health partnerships. As the environments of hospitals have changed, questions arise as to how the roles and functions of trustees must change to better serve their organizations and communities. Indeed, in the popular literature, there is growing sentiment that the role of hospital trustees will become increasingly central to hospital effectiveness and survival. It has been argued that the functions of governance are broadening, that trustees have become accountable for hospital performance and community health, and that the trustee role is becoming more complex and demanding. Hospital governance is being required to develop and oversee organizational policy that reflects multiple and often conflicting pressures emanating from social imperatives, public expectations, community need, cost control, quality improvement and assurance, and technological development.

In fact, these pronouncements and predictions have been based largely on speculation and anecdotal information rather than careful analysis. More fundamental concerns about whether boards and trustees are catalysts for change or, alternatively, sources of stability or even barriers to adaptation require careful systematic examination. The purpose of this chapter is to propose a framework for thinking about some of the likely changes in the role and function of hospital trustees, drawing where possible on recent research to inform the discussion.

CAN HOSPITAL GOVERNANCE ADAPT?

Why should we assume that trustee roles and responsibilities need to change, even in the face of sea changes in the hospital environment? After all, the fundamental functions of hospital trustees might be seen as enduring ones—fulfilling fiduciary responsibilities, overseeing management, ensuring quality of care, and representing the community interest in hospital policymaking.[1] We know historically, however, that the role of trustees has changed over time, largely as a function of shifts in funding and power held by various stakeholders in the health care arena, and the consequent changes in the role of the hospital itself. For example, in the mid- to late-nineteenth century, hospital trustees made many decisions now thought to be the province of medical professionals, such as admitting and discharging patients. Such responsibilities were directly linked to the rudimentary state of medical knowledge at the time, the need for community legitimacy, and the pressing need for working capital. From these needs resulted an organizational structure—in private as well as public hospitals—in which boards of "managers," trustees, governors or commissioners, rather than physicians or professional administrators, retained final decision-making power.[2]

Over the years, the role of the hospital trustee has shifted with the development of medical knowledge and technology, the commensurate rise in physician power and, most recently, the growing complexity of the health care economic and regulatory environment. The key point here is that the very notion of trusteeship and governance has changed as the role and function of the hospital itself have changed. It seems opportune, in this era of rapid upheaval in the health care industry, to begin to think about how these changes might have an impact on the role of the hospital trustee and how the existing state of knowledge / research on hospital trusteeship can inform our perspective on these issues.

THE STATE OF RESEARCH ON HOSPITAL GOVERNANCE AND TRUSTEESHIP

A second issue is related to how research on hospital governance can help us understand the likely changes that trusteeship will experience in the coming years. The state of research, though improving, is not robust and must be used with caution to inform our discussion of the changing roles of hospital trustee. There simply is not a critical mass of empirical research in the area of health care governance that can be used to guide practice. And that which does exist has not established a consistent relationship between governance and other outcomes of interest (e.g., hospital effectiveness).[3]

In many respects, the ambiguity surrounding hospital board roles and functions is reflected in the management and research literature on health care organizations. Economic models of hospitals, for example, have typically viewed the hospital organization as essentially a physician cooperative.[4] Under this view, boards serve only to legitimize the hospital in the community and the larger society. Others have employed an exchange perspective, in which the only relevant actors in the hospital are managers and medical staff.[5] Most comparative studies of hospital decision making also have failed to examine the influence of trustees in relation to other groups within the institution, such as managers and the medical staff. Implicitly, these studies have assumed that trustees and governing boards were either ineffectual or of marginal importance as an internal decision-making body. The problems above notwithstanding, there is an emerging body of research on hospital and corporate governance upon which we will draw to selectively support arguments related to the changing roles of hospital trustees. This work is primarily descriptive, but it has the advantage of tracking change in governing boards and trustees over time, an attribute well suited to our present task.

HOSPITAL INSTITUTIONAL CHANGE

There has been an enormous volume of writing on the fundamental forces at work to change the strategic context, incentives, and regulatory / payment structure under which hospitals operate. I will not attempt to replicate these writings here. Interestingly, much less has been written about the fundamental ways in which hospitals (and, by extension, trustees) have responded to these fundamental shifts.[6] There are five broad institutional responses that have defined hospital organizational change in the past ten to fifteen years. These issues have also been instrumental in shaping research on hospital trusteeship during this period and, not surprisingly, the questions about roles and functions of trustees in a changing health care context. Each of these five changes will be discussed and followed by an analysis of the implications of the changes for hospital trusteeship.

The first, "consolidation," refers to a range of organizational restructuring activities designed to position hospitals to take advantage of scale economies and/or complementarity in services, personnel, or markets. Often, consolidation is associated with combining the assets of two or more previously independent organizations. However, consolidation can also include the elimination of hospital capacity when redundancy in a system or market occurs. Examples of consolidation include the formation of health care systems (horizontally and vertically integrated), network formation, hospital mergers, closures, and conversions of acute care hospitals to other forms of health care delivery. Recent data indicate that fully 50 percent of all hospitals are members of a health care system and another 39 percent are participants in some form of network arrangement with other organizations.

The second general response to the sea changes being experienced by the health care sector can be termed "the search for efficiency." Under the Diagnosis Related Group system of reimbursement and, more recently, under pressure from managed care organizations and employer groups, hospitals have turned their attention inward to improve operating systems. Health care payers, specifically, are immediately affected by rising costs and have demanded that hospitals provide care at a lower cost. In practice, this means that hospitals must find ways of improving the efficiencies with which care is delivered—a concern that is relatively new in the field. For example, under capitated reimbursement, hospital financial viability will be a direct function of the degree to which care can be provided for a cost below the capitated rate. Hospital management, once concerned primarily with managing external relations with regulators, payers, and other stakeholders, must now focus its attention equally on issues of downsizing, appropriate balance between primary care and specialists on the medial staff, and perhaps most important, redesigning the internal operating systems of the organization.[7]

The third response by hospitals has been "the search for value." In some respects, this response may be viewed as a reaction to the perceived overemphasis on cost containment and efficiency that pervades public policy discussions and competitive dynamics in the health care sector. Questions are being raised, for example, about the lengths to which hospitals should go in reducing costs. Should these efficiencies come at the price of quality reduction or diminution of community service? More emphasis is now being placed on striking the appropriate balance between efficiency and quality. In many cases, hospitals are engaged in designing clinical protocols, pathways, or best practices that simultaneously control excessive costs while at the same time reducing undesired variability in treatment outcomes. In practical terms, this means that hospitals are required to form new relationships with their affiliated physicians. The traditional arm's-length approach of the past is no longer viable when active dialogue and partnership are required to merge the interests of quality and cost containment.[8] Active physician membership in hospital management and governance has been on the rise, as have tighter forms of integration between hospitals and physicians.[9] This can take the form of group practices sponsored or owned by the hospital, the purchase of physician practices, or more complex intermediate forms of organization that link hospitals and physician groups (e.g., physician–hospital organizations).

The fourth institutional response by hospitals takes the form of "alliance building." Alliances are nonhierarchical forms of organizing that are voluntary in nature and that depend on the interdependence among participants. As health care delivery becomes more complex and costly, more organizations are realizing that they lack the resources, expertise, or market presence to "go it alone." The development of strategic partnerships—designed to gain market footholds, forestall competitors' moves, or fill critical gaps in core competencies—are becoming increasingly common among hospitals and other types of delivery organizations. These virtual organizations are structured and managed very differently from the traditional hierarchically based organizations and, indeed, require different skills to operate and sustain them. Issues of accountability, balancing competing demands, and avoiding turf battles are but a few of the thorny problems encountered in making alliances work.[10] Despite these problems, alliances offer considerable potential advantages to hospitals that lack all the requisite tools to successfully compete in today's market. They are flexible and are capable of being expanded or reduced depending on need. They are less costly than more capital-intensive forms of organization, and they promote cooperation, an approach to health care delivery that has received too little attention in an era of competition and managed care.

The fifth and final institutional response by health care organizations is the "development of integrated health care systems (IHS)." Integrated health care systems are multiorganizational arrangements designed to provide a wide range of health and preventive services across the continuum of care. Typically, IHS combine the physician and the functional and clinical components of care delivery in a manner to control appropriate access, utilization, and quality of services for patients or members of a health plan.[11] As with the other forms of institutional response, IHS offer many potential advantages in an environment that emphasizes cost control, access, and a full spectrum of services that are appropriately coordinated. Proponents of IHS maintain that these organizational forms rationalize the delivery of care, reduce fragmentation, and reduce the inherently conflicting incentives that pervade the health care delivery system. The emergence of these complex systems, however, is not without detractors who claim that they are cumbersome, incapable of adapting quickly to market changes, expensive to manage and operate, and slow in producing their promised results.[12]

MAJOR THEMES IN CURRENT HOSPITAL GOVERNANCE RESEARCH

These five broad institutional responses to fundamental shifts in the health care sector have also informed the research questions on health care governance during the past ten to fifteen years. To the extent that hospital boards and trustees are ultimately responsible for the viability and strategic direction of the organizations they govern, the conceptual and empirical links between institutional response and governance seem logical. This research can be classified into five major streams. The first is concerned with issues of how boards relate to higher authorities, and centers on the themes of accountability, decision-making control, and power in new organizational arrangements.[13] As hospitals become components of larger systems and more complex organizational structures, the notion of the board as an independent decision-making body, accountable exclusively to the community, is rapidly being called into question. Multiple forms of accountability—to the community, to corporate entities, to other system organizations—are now the norm. How the board manages these accountabilities and which entity should hold decision-making authority are the two dominant themes in writing on governance.

Specifically, potential conflicts engendered by multiple agency roles make designing appropriate incentives, compensation, and evaluation systems a high priority for governance and trustees. Research in this area also tells us that the appropriate locus of control in a health care system depends on the decision in question, as well as the attributes of the system itself (e.g., geographic dispersion, size).[14] For example, the local hospital board often makes quality improvement decisions while governing bodies at the corporate level make capital allocation decisions. The primary contribution of this body of research is to illuminate the fact that hospital boards and trustees operate in a more complex, interconnected world and that the roles and functions of trustees must be reevaluated in the context of the system in which they operate.

A second major stream of research centers on the question of governance and organizational performance. As hospitals and health care systems are becoming increasingly concerned about their performance in the market and their accountability to health plans, there has been a commensurate emphasis on evaluating the performance contributions of organizational systems (including governance). The research question dominating this area "is what difference does governance make in organizational success and/or viability?" This stream of research, for example, examines the relationship between board composition and hospital financial performance, or the association between board structure and major organizational/strategic change.[15] Findings from this research indicate that board leadership (particularly from physicians) is instrumental in achieving positive financial performance and effective implementation of quality improvement initiatives. On the whole, however, the hospital and health services literature on governing boards and performance does not reach any consistent conclusions regarding the relationships between board characteristics and hospital effectiveness. A major contribution of this literature to date is the identification and classification of observed differences in types of boards.[16]

Board–management relations constitute the third area of governance research. Here the fundamental questions concern how the board exercises its agency role as a guardian of the community interest while balancing the need for closer cooperation with management. Traditionally, hospital boards and management have been quite separate, with many hospitals not permitting managers to serve on the board, much less as an active voting member. However, the changing competitive and regulatory climate has afforded managers greater power over hospital affairs and a more active role in the governance process. These closer ties have, in the eyes of some, compromised the ability of the board to effectively exercise its agency role in ensuring that management acts in a way consistent with the interests of the community. Indeed, much of the discussion about the relative merits of the corporate model of governance has centered on the role of the organizational chief executive officer (CEO) on the board.[17] Research in this area has examined the incentive, compensation, evaluation, and contractual relations between the board and hospital management in relation to specific behavioral (e.g., turnover) and performance outcomes. One of the key contributions of this stream of research has been to describe the substitutability of various agency mechanisms for different types of hospitals and to reveal unintended (negative) consequences of specific types of control systems (e.g., contracts) for management behavior. For example, research has shown that the use of formal employment contracts for hospital CEOs results in greater instability in that position.[18]

The fourth area of research in hospital governance has been concerned with the evolutionary development of board roles. This research assumes that the role and functions of hospital boards are not static but change over time and with different contingencies that hospitals face in their growth and development. This research has shown, for example, that many boards assume a passive role during periods of market prosperity and stability but take a more activist posture during periods of crisis or environmental instability. Others have pointed to the symbolic functions assumed by trustees and hospital boards in reinforcing the ideals of volunteerism and local control in hospital affairs, although exercising little in the way of actual operational or policy influence in such matters.[19] By contrast, some have noted the inappropriate operational roles assumed by some trustees. These activities are assumed to be antithetical to board roles and inconsistent with the policymaking and oversight functions normally assumed by hospital boards.

A contribution of this stream of research is to highlight that the roles and functions of boards may vary under different operating conditions and/or evolutionary periods in hospital development and that boards will differ in their roles, responsibilities, and functions across different types of hospitals. By extension, this research argues that it may be dangerous to assume that all boards and trustees should be doing the same thing or provide similar value to the institutions they govern. Another way of conceptualizing the multiplicity of board roles is to consider the value of governance in trusteeship from the perspective of different hospital stakeholders. For example, management may view the board as a partner in effecting strategic change, while the community may see the board's role as emphasizing community interest and need. Other stakeholders—such as regulatory bodies, payers, and society as a whole—may view still different functions as paramount for the board.[20]

The final, and perhaps newest, area of research focuses on configurational analysis of boards and board structures. Increasingly, scholars now view hospital governing boards as consisting of a series of interconnected and highly interdependent components rather than as a set of independent elements that can be effectively separated from each other. This research examines how different elements of board structure, composition, and process fit together as a system. A recent example documented how hospital boards are moving toward what scholars refer to as a corporate model of governance, and the conditions under which hospitals are likely to adopt such corporate governance configurations.[21] Corporate governance is seen as a set of interrelated components that emphasize a small number of trustees, focus on highly selected skills or backgrounds of trustees, perform tight evaluation or scrutiny of the CEO, expect greater management participation on the board, and place more emphasis on strategic concerns of the hospital. This research has served to refocus attention on the gestalt of governance and its many elements as opposed to narrowly focusing on one element (e.g., board size, term limits for board members). This work has also served to reinforce the notion that governing bodies are like organizations themselves and consist of many different facets, all of which have to work together as a system to be effective.

IMPLICATIONS FOR GOVERNANCE AND TRUSTEESHIP

The areas of research discussed above give rise to a number of different issues and questions regarding the role of trustees in the future, and the challenges that these trustees might face in a changing health care environment. Broadly speaking, these issues can be divided into four major subgroups: (1) the embeddedness of governance systems, (2) board–management relations, (3) the emergence of new organizational forms, and (4) the new work of trustees.

The embeddedness of governance systems suggests that the era of the free-standing hospital board, and independent board of trustees, is rapidly becoming a thing of the past. Increasingly, organizational providers, including hospitals, operate within the context of larger organizational systems. Recent data suggest that 40 to 60 percent of all hospitals now operate as part of a larger health care system or network. These networks or systems might include multi-hospital systems, integrated health care systems, university hospitals, or various forms of alliances or networks. Hospital participation in these multilayered organizational forms adds a new level of complexity to governance, one that potentially makes hospital trustees accountable, or at least responsive, to the interests and concerns of other organizational boards or superordinate authorities. Increasingly, the field has begun to replace the notion of institutional governance with the idea of systems of governance. Health care systems, for example, are increasingly concerned with not only how effectively individual boards operate but also with how well the system of governance operates. The latter might focus on the communication among different boards within the same system, the division of decision-making authority and responsibility within the governance system, and the limits of local versus corporate control over system policymaking and operations.

Three specific issues are raised under governance embeddedness. The first issue is the changes in the roles and functions of trustees in governance systems. Traditionally, governing boards have been focused on the hospital as an institution and the local community as the accountable entity. Under a more complex, embedded governance structure, questions are raised as to who is responsible for what. For example, should the local board be primarily responsible for quality assurance and CEO evaluation while boards at the system level take responsibility for capital allocation and broader strategic decisions? Similarly, should the primary mission of the local hospital board be to ensure that the hospital remains competitive in its local market, while operating within the broad strategic or mission guidelines of the system?

The second issue raised by governance embeddedness relates to accountability. Specifically, to what entity does the local board owe its primary allegiance—the community, the system, or to other organizational entities that are also members of the system? The challenge in an embedded governance system will be to balance the various reporting relationships and accountabilities to effectively meet the needs of all stakeholders involved. This will be no mean feat given that the interest of the community, for example, may differ from the broader strategic goals of the system in which the hospital is embedded.

The third and final issue under governance embeddedness stems from the nature of the interlocking structures that define the system of governance. With increasingly complex systems, the challenges for governance are also increased. Many systems will wish to consider consolidating their multiple governing bodies to streamline decision making. This may consist of the elimination of local boards entirely, the substitution of advisory boards for local governing boards, or the creation of regional governing bodies in lieu of organizational or institutionally focused boards.[22] The second way in which governance complexities in systems may be managed is through compositional changes of boards. One of the key challenges of a governance system will be the way in which multiple boards communicate with each other, and the extent to which they can work independently within a broad, common framework. A common strategy for realizing these objectives is to ensure cross membership on boards within the system, as well as representation by key partner organizations on the boards of local hospitals. This board-interlock strategy is common in the corporate sector, and we may see it used with increasing frequency in health care systems.

Governing boards and trustees would be well advised, however, to recognize that such interlock strategies often come at a price. For example, representation on the system board by local governing board members may result in a parochial orientation to the interests of the local operating entities, rather than the broader goals of the system.[23] Such costs should be weighed with the potential advantages of obtaining needed information about local market conditions and the operating unit.

A second set of issues emerging from the literature on hospital governance relates to new forms of board management relations. Traditionally, there has been a separation of board and management in hospitals. Hospital boards have essentially been community boards, consisting primarily of outside members of the community who exercise oversight over hospital management and who communicate the needs of community through board meetings or personal relations with hospital management. Many have raised questions regarding how the board should relate to management in an era of competition and rapid change. Some are calling for closer working relations and a greater role for management on hospital boards to make the board more adaptive and responsive to changing market conditions, and to reduce the decision-making cycle time. Indeed, data from recent surveys on hospital governance suggest that board–management relations are the area of governance most likely to have exhibited change during the past ten years.

Three specific issues are raised under the heading of board–management relations. The first is the identification of management roles vis-à-vis the board. What should management's role be on the board? Should he or she serve as a voting member, an observer, or should he or she chair the board? Should other members of the management team, such as the chief financial officer or chief legal officer, be included in the governance process? Clearly, greater insider participation on boards potentially changes the basic relationship between management and governance to one of partnership. At the same time, it raises specific concerns about the ability of the board to fulfill its traditional agency role of monitoring management and ensuring that the hospital performs in the community's best interest.

Indeed, the second major issue raised by changing board–management relations is how the board and its trustees fulfill their agency roles in the context of closer working relations with management. We know from our data that along with closer management–board relations, there is also a commensurate increase in accountability mechanisms exercised by the board. For example, there has been an increasing use of formal employment contracts between the board and hospital CEOs, increased use of incentive compensation packages for the CEO, as well as more extensive use of formal performance evaluations of the CEO.

The third and final issue raised by changing board–management relations relates directly to the shifting power balance between physicians and managers. Increasingly, trustees are being placed in the position where they must mediate between the potentially conflicting interest of physicians and managers as both respond to changing market demands imposed by managed care firms, large employers, and changing regulatory requirements. These changing conditions have increased the amount of instability between management and medical staff but, at the same time, provided opportunities for new forms of relationships and increased incentives for alignment of strategic and economic interests between the two groups.[24] Often, it falls to the board to identify these opportunities for alignment and to ensure that both groups are working toward a common set of goals and the greater good. This suggests that a primary role of trustees in the future will be to clearly communicate the vision for the organization and to ensure that all parties (internal and external) engage in strategies to ultimately achieve that vision.

The third area arising from the research literature on governance is the emergence of new organizational forms in the health care sector. With increased emphasis on competition and the lowering of regulatory barriers in most states (e.g., Certificate of Need regulations, rate review), barriers to entry and exit to health care markets have been effectively removed. Coupled with an increase in competition, this has resulted in a burgeoning of new organizational entities within the health care sector. These include vertically integrated systems, specialized service providers, various forms of managed care organizations, and perhaps most pertinent to this discussion, alliances and networks as forms of organizing health care delivery. Many of these new organizations are shifting from a narrow, institutional focus on the hospital, or on hospital care, to a broader strategic focus that includes an emphasis on prevention, care for enrolled populations, and improving the health of the community at large.

Further, many of these new organizational forms have nonhierarchically based structures that depend on trust and common vision among members of the alliance or partnership. Traditional agency relationships are blurred insofar as members of the partnership or alliance have a loyalty not only to the partnership but also to their individual home organizations. These dual interests may correspond or differ by degree as well as over time. The absence of rigid reporting relationships and formal organizational structures contribute to making the task of governance more ambiguous than it is in typical hospital settings.

The governance of partnerships and alliances requires a very different conceptual orientation to management, governance, and leadership than has been present in traditional hierarchically based organizations. First, the notion of mutuality is paramount. It is essential for the survival and well-being of partnerships and alliances that there be a win–win situation among members of a partnership; each participant must feel that they have something to gain by participating. Further, it is important for governance to ensure that a strong sense of interdependence among partnership members is achieved. If partner members feel that they are no longer benefiting from their association with other partners, then there is no reason for them to continue to participate. This rather fragile basis of partnerships and networks is decidedly different from the more hierarchically and inducement-based foundations that characterize hospitals. Governing boards and trustees must be sensitive to these differences if they are to exercise effective oversight over these entities.

A second principle characterizing strategic alliances and health partnerships is that it is not necessary that all partners receive equal benefits from participating. The principle of equity rather than equality among partners should be a basic operating premise. That is, partner organizations do not have to receive an equal share of the benefits of partnership participation, but they do need to receive benefits consistent with their contributions, and their views have to be considered and respected, regardless of their contribution. Learning how to strike this delicate balance will be a new task for many trustees and governing boards.

Finally, boards and trustees must recognize that in many cases they will be cooperating and competing with other organizations simultaneously. In the context of a competitive health care environment, there is room for both coop-eration and competition. Clearly, a key role of trustees will be to recognize and differentiate those situations in which competition is appropriate from those in which the organizations should cooperate. Again, this requires trustees to think very differently about strategy, policymaking, and external relations.

These and other developments have raised issues about the decision-making responsibilities of boards and trustees and have led to a reconsideration of how boards should actually carry out their responsibilities in a vastly different health care context. For example, whereas trustees have been traditionally concerned with issues of the quality of care in the hospital, they are now being asked to define quality in very different ways than they have in the past. More emphasis is being placed on quality improvement and the board's role in providing lead-ership in efforts to improve clinical care at a reasonable cost. Similarly, the notion of quality is now being extended beyond simply the quality of care pro-vided to patients in inpatient settings. Increasingly, hospital boards will be asked to consider population-level quality indicators that are reflective of the health status of the community as a whole, and developing appropriate bench-marks to gauge the hospital's contribution to improving those quality stan-dards. In a sense, we continue to use the old terminology with which boards and trustees have long been familiar, but these terms have taken on radically new meanings in the new health care environment.

Other types of decisions and functions will be unchanged but will require increasing scrutiny and emphasis on the part of trustees. In particular, the focus on values and vision for the organization becomes more salient in times of rapid change and uncertainty. Hospital CEOs will come and go, but trustees are the institutional anchor of the hospital. They provide continuity in uphold-ing the long-term goals of the organization, as well as continuity in reinforcing the values that support that vision. Finally, the decisions that hospital boards and trustees will have to make will focus increasingly on how to take the orga-nization into the future rather than reviewing what has occurred in the past month or since the last board meeting. Focusing on immediate past perfor-mance will place the institution at great risk unless these "reporting out" con-cerns are balanced by a serious consideration of the needs of the institution in the future. This can take the form of strategic planning, scenario building, or simply a thoughtful discussion of where the hospital wants to be in the next ten to fifteen years.

THE NEW WORK OF TRUSTEES

To engage in these new types of decisions, and to preserve the viability of the hospital in the future, the board and its trustees must redefine its work. Whereas the environment in health care in the past forty years has been particularly forgiving of mistakes and tolerant of lack of attention to future needs, this is no longer the case. The work of boards and trustees cannot be simply focused on preserving the assets of the organization. The new work of boards must, first and foremost, be concerned with the crucial do-or-die issues central to the hospital's success.[25] This can take the form of strategy making, developing and promulgating organizational values, or dealing with the positioning of the hospital in a rapidly changing and highly competitive health care marketplace. It does *not* mean reviewing in great detail operational issues or financial details provided since the last board meeting.

A second element of the new work of boards is that it is driven by results linked to defined timetables. This means working within a plan, not simply vague promises provided by management. The board must be ruthless in insisting that management carry out its strategies and work toward its vision in a systematic, concrete way.

Consistent with the need for a defined timetable is the requirement that quantifiable measures of success be provided to, or be developed by, the board. This means that the board should emphasize appropriate data and strive to be knowledgeable, particularly on issues of strategy, long-term policy, and achieving the vision of the organization. It also means, by contrast, that the board not deal with data that are irrelevant to these broad, crucial issues, and that it spends its time reviewing information that would allow it to make more informed decisions about these central concerns.

Finally, the new work of boards requires specific engagement of the hospital's internal and external constituencies. Moving organizations into the future requires an understanding and concerted effort on the part of all parties— employees, physicians, management, regulators, customers, and payers. A key function of trustees in the future will be to ensure that there is no imbalance in the attention being paid to one stakeholder group at the expense of another. The board and its trustees, in other words, will operate at a critical nexus, uniquely positioned to engage all stakeholders necessary to define the vision of the organization and to carry it forward into the future.

TRANSITION TO NEW GOVERNANCE ROLES

If hospital governing boards and their trustees choose to embrace these new roles and decisions, how will they make the transition between traditional structures and roles and the new models of governance? I propose seven guidelines for managing the governance transition to new roles and responsibilities. The first focuses on a conceptual reorientation toward trusteeship that supplements traditional fiduciary responsibilities and an orientation toward preserving the assets of the hospital. Trustees must simply learn to think about governance in a very different light in view of the many changes that are being experienced by the health care sector and the hospital industry.

Of course, this will not be an easy undertaking, and it must be reinforced by the second and third transition guidelines—ongoing education and shared learning. Ongoing education refers to providing the board and its trustees with "on-the-job" exposure to high-quality information about changes in the health care sector and their implications for the institutions they govern. This may take the form of off-site retreats, presentations by external consultants, or carefully selected reading material. The key is that this should be an ongoing and institutionalized component of the governance process, not something that occurs on an annual or less frequent basis.

Shared learning refers to the creation of synergies between trustees and management, or trustees and external stakeholders, through the sharing of information and ideas. Clearly, the hierarchical form of oversight traditionally performed by boards may be experiencing rapid obsolescence owing to the pace of change and the complexity of issues facing boards and the institutions they govern. An orientation toward a true exchange of knowledge and learning can increase the quality of governance decisions and serve to involve key internal and external stakeholders, indicating a common vision for the hospital.

The fourth guideline centers on establishing the vision of the organization as the centerpiece of the board and its activities. As was stated above, in an era of constant flux and change, having a clear vision of where the organization wants to be in the future will be an important sustaining vehicle for employees, governing-board members, and management. It is a primary responsibility of the board to clarify that vision and communicate it effectively to all parties. It should be used as a guideline for virtually all decisions made by the board and the basis for conducting oversight of management.

The fifth guideline involves introducing appropriate incentives to change. Trustees can exhort management to move the hospital in the direction of the vision, but in practical terms this requires that appropriate incentive structures be put in place to ensure that those behaviors are in fact realized. The board may wish to carefully review the nature of contracts, financial incentive systems, and/or formal evaluation in monitoring systems to make them consistent with the long-term goals of the organization. Often boards operate on inertia and historical precedent rather than attempting to achieve a fit between these incentives for change and the goals of this change.

The sixth guideline for transition relates to the board's relationship with the community that they represent. Clearly, as the focus of health care organizations shifts from treating patients who are admitted to the hospital to serving the needs of the community and enhancing the health of that community, input on the part of community members who are being served needs to be more direct and immediate. Boards need to actively consider how to expand community involvement in the governance process or alternatively how the governance process can be extended to reach out into the community in order to assess community needs and to ensure that the hospital is doing all it can to meet those needs.

Finally, change in governance and in governance practices can be best accomplished if boards and their trustees have a means of keeping score. By this I mean the introduction of systematic data collection, benchmarking and milestones available to trustees to ensure that they can monitor not only when the vision has been achieved, or when ultimate goals have been accomplished, but also the extent to which intermediate goals have been met. This will require careful consideration on the part of both management and trustees in developing a set of meaningful but limited indicators that reflect the progress of the institution toward its vision and goals. At the same time, organizations should eliminate extraneous or irrelevant information presented to the board that would distract it from its primary purpose.

There is little doubt that hospitals and hospital trustees will be affected by the profound changes that are occurring in the health care sector. These changes have led to new issues, problems, uncertainties, and opportunities for hospital boards and trustees. In addition to the fundamental market and regulatory shifts that are creating radically different incentives for hospital behavior, trustees must continue to confront traditionally thorny issues, including responding to competitive pressures from other hospitals and, increasingly, physician groups; maintaining the delicate balance between physicians as competitors and physicians as partners; increased scrutiny of both clinical and operational quality; and the many ethical dilemmas related to the provision of charity care, discontinuance of services, and end-of-life decisions.

These changes compel the hospital board and its trustees to play more active roles not only in organizational affairs but also, more broadly, in ensuring accountability to the communities in which the hospital operates. At an individual level, trustees must exhibit a wide range of skills and perspectives, ranging from finance and insurance to legal and strategic management. Hospital trustees must be able to both react to and anticipate emerging issues and problems in a highly volatile marketplace and health-sector environment. Hospital trustees are, accordingly, shifting their orientation to changing rather than maintaining the status quo. Often this may entail restructuring relationships between the hospital and the larger system to which it belongs, or its role in a heath care alliance or network. Even traditional concepts that have represented the foundation of hospital trusteeship in the past are being reconsidered, most notably, trustees' orientation to the community and their agency role vis-à-vis management.

Much of the writing in this chapter has been prescriptive. However, it is important to note that changes are occurring in governing boards and among trustees differently for different types of hospitals. For example, investor-owned hospitals tend to foster physician participation on their governing boards more aggressively than do public and private not-for-profit hospitals. The boards of larger hospitals are far more likely to use a formal self-evaluation process than smaller hospitals.

These and the many other types of differences between types of hospitals point to the importance of avoiding a one-size-fits-all approach to hospital governance and change in trusteeship. Executives, board members, external experts, policymakers, consultants, and researchers must take into consideration the specific organizational and environmental characteristics in which the hospital operates. Just as there are appropriate fits between organizational strategy and market characteristics, there also should be a fit between governance structures and functions and the nature of the organization being governed. Inappropriate comparisons across types of hospitals should be avoided. For example, it may be unrealistic to expect small rural hospitals to have large numbers of physicians on their boards when physicians in rural areas tend to be scarce, their time completely filled with patient care activities, and their ability to leverage decision making already largely on a personal basis. Similarly, one should not expect public hospitals to emulate the governance practices of investor-owned or even private not-for-profit hospitals: They typically face different legislative restraints, accountability arrangements, and public funding features than do other hospitals.

NOTES

1. M. L. Fennell and J. A. Alexander, "Governing Boards and Profound Organizational Change in Hospitals," *Medical Care Review* 46, no. 2 (1989): 157–87.

2. P. Starr, *The Social Transformation of American Medicine* (New York: Basic Books, 1982).

3. J. A. Alexander and H. S. Zuckerman, "Health Care Governance: Are We Keeping Pace?" *Journal of Health Administration Education* 7 (1989): 760–77.

4. M. Pauly and M. Redisch, "The Not-for-Profit Hospital as a Physician's Cooperative," *American Economic Review* 63 (1973): 87–99.

5. P. Jacobs, "A Survey of Economic Models of Hospitals," *Inquiry* 11 (1974): 83–97; J. F. Harris, *The New Industrial State* (New York: New American Library, 1977).

6. Harris, *New Industrial State*.

7. American Hospital Association, *AHA Guide to the Health Care Field* (Chicago: American Hospital Association, 1998).

8. B. J. Weiner, J. A. Alexander, and S. Shortell, "Leadership for Quality Improvement in Health Care: Empirical Evidence on Hospital Boards, Managers, and Physicians," *Medical Care Research and Review* 53, no. 4 (1996): 397–416; B. J. Weiner and J. A. Alexander, "Hospital

Governance and Quality of Care: A Critical Review of Transitional Roles," *Medical Care Review* 50, no. 4 (1993): 375–410.

9. J. A. Alexander, L. R. Burns, H. S. Zuckerman, T. Vaughn, R. M. Andersen, P. Torrens, and D. W. Hilberman, "An Exploratory Analysis of Market-Based, Physician-Organization Arrangements," *Hospital and Health Services Administration* 41, no. 3 (1996): 311–29; J. A. Alexander, T. Vaughn, L. R. Burns, H. S. Zuckerman, R. M. Anderson, P. Torrens, and D. W. Hilberman, "Organizational Approaches to Integrated Health Care Delivery: A Taxonomic Analysis of Physician-Organization Arrangements," *Medical Care Research and Review* 53, no. 1 (1996): 70–93.

10. B. J. Weiner and J. A. Alexander, "The Challenges of Governing Public–Private Community Health Partnerships," *Health Care Management Review* 23, no. 2 (1998): 39–55.

11. S. M. Shortell, R. R. Gillies, D. A. Anderson, K. Morgan-Erickson, and J. B. Mitchell, *Remaking Health Care in America: Building Organized Delivery Systems* (San Francisco: Jossey-Bass, 1996).

12. S. Mick and Associates, *Innovations in Health Care Delivery: Insights for Organization Theory* (Ann Arbor, Mich.: Health Administration Press, 1990); L. R. Burns and J. Robinson, "Physician Practice Management Companies: Implications for Hospital-Based Integrated Delivery Systems," *Frontiers of Health Services Management* 14, no. 2 (1997): 3–35.

13. L. Morlock and J. A. Alexander, "Models of Governance in Multihospital Systems: Implications for Hospital and System-Level Decision Making," *Medical Care* 24, no. 12 (1986): 1118–35; J. A. Alexander, L. Morlock, and B. Gifford, "The Effects of Corporate Restructuring on Hospital Policymaking," *Health Services Research* 23, no. 2 (1988): 311–27; M. L. Fennell and J. A. Alexander, "Organizational Boundary-Spanning and Institutionalized Environments," *Academy of Management Journal* 30, no. 3 (1987): 456–76.

14. J. A. Alexander and M. L. Fennell, "Patterns of Decision Making in Multihospital Systems," *Journal of Health and Social Behavior* 27, no. 1 (1986): 14–27; J. A. Alexander, "Hospital Governance: Problems and Prospects for Health Services Research," *Journal of Health Administration Education* 9, no. 4 (1991): 395–424.

15. C. Molinari, L. Morlock, J. A. Alexander, and C. A. Lyles, "Hospital Board Effectiveness: Relationships between Governing Board Composition and Hospital Financial Viability," *Health Services Research* 28, no. 3 (1993): 357–77; Fennell and Alexander, "Governing Boards"; B. J. Weiner, S. Shortell, and J. A. Alexander, "Promoting Clinical Involvement in Hospital Quality Improvement Efforts: The Effects of Top Management, Board, and Physician Leadership," *Health Services Research* 32, no. 4 (1997): 491–510.

16. B. J. Weiner and J. A. Alexander, "Corporate and Philanthropic Models of Hospital Governance: A Taxonomic Evaluation," *Health Services Research* 28, no. 3 (1993): 325–55.

17. Weiner and Alexander, "Corporate and Philanthropic Models"; J. A. Alexander and B. J. Weiner, "The Adoption of the Corporate Governance Model by Nonprofit Organizations," *Non-Profit Management and Leadership* 8, no. 3 (1998): 223–42.

18. J. A. Alexander, M. L. Fennell, and M. T. Halpern, "Leadership Instability in Hospitals: The Influence of Board–CEO Relations and Organizational Growth and Decline," *Administrative Science Quarterly* 38 (1993): 74–99.

19. D. Starkweather, "Hospital Board Power," *Health Services Management Research* 1, no. 27 (1988): 74–86; J. A. Alexander, *The Changing Character of Hospital Governance* (Chicago: Hospital Research and Educational Trust, 1990).

20. J. A. Alexander, "Governance for Whom? Dilemmas of Change and Effectiveness in Hospital Boards," *Frontiers of Health Services Management* 6, no. 3 (1990): 38–41; M. N. Zald, "The Power and Function of Boards of Directors: A Theoretical Synthesis," *American Journal of Sociology* 75 (1969): 97–111.

21. Alexander and Weiner, "Adoption of the Corporate Governance Model."

22. D. D. Pointer, J. A. Alexander, and H. S. Zuckerman, "Loosening the Gordian Knot of Governance in Integrated Health Care Delivery Systems," *Frontiers of Health Services Management* 11, no. 3 (1995): 3–37; reprinted in *Integrated Delivery Systems: Creation, Management and Governance* (Chicago: Health Administration Press, 1997).

23. Pointer, Alexander, and Zuckerman, "Loosening the Gordian Knot."

24. K. G. Provan, "Organizational and Decision Unit Characteristics and Board Influence in Independent versus Multihospital System-Affiliated Hospitals," *Journal of Health and Social Behavior* 29 (1988): 239–52; Alexander, "Hospital Governance."

25. R. P. Chait, *The Effective Board of Trustees* (New York: American Council on Education and Oryx Press, 1991).

4

THE ROLE OF HOSPITALS IN THE COMMUNITY

Romana Hasnain-Wynia, Frances S. Margolin,
and Mary A. Pittman

During the past century, hospitals have evolved from organizations providing acute care services to sick patients into complex modern health care systems supporting a wide range of initiatives. One thing that has not changed, however, is the role of the hospital as a major asset in its community. Today there are many examples of hospitals focusing on improving the health care and health status of citizens in their local communities. More and more, hospitals are making strategic use of their financial, human, and technical resources to strengthen the ability of local communities to support and sustain community health. In many small cities and towns, the hospital is one of the major employers and economic engines. In larger cities, within geographic or culturally defined communities, it may serve as a key safety net provider of care for underserved populations. The hospital trustee's role is critical in preserving these assets and facilitating the commitment to community health.

However, increased pressures in the past decade have challenged the role of the hospital within the community and that of the trustee. These are due, in part, to decreased government reimbursement, stringent managed care contracts, personnel shortages, Health Portability and Accountability Act (HIPAA) regulations, and mergers and de-mergers. Trustees have increasingly had to focus on the financial well-being of the institution rather than the role of the hospital in the broader community, thus creating a tension as to the trustee's primary role and responsibilities. Despite environmental and other strains, there remains the significant role that hospitals play and that trustees steward— the role of supporting and sustaining community health. Through collaboration with other community organizations, many hospitals focus on improving not just health, strictly defined, but also quality of life—that is, health in its broadest definition: Health is the state of complete physical, mental, and social well-being and not merely the absence of disease or infirmity.[1]

This chapter presents reasons why a hospital should address questions of community and population health, looks at how hospitals work with other organizations in their communities to do so, and discusses how hospitals sustain their commitment to community health in the face of financial pressures. It also discusses the role of trustees in promoting and sustaining that commitment.

WHY ADDRESS COMMUNITY HEALTH?

One model for hospital–community collaboration is the Community Care Network (CCN).[2] Since the mid-1990s, the American Hospital Association's Health Research and Educational Trust has served as the national program office for the CCN demonstration program, which consists of twenty-five public–private partnerships around the country.[3] Each of these partnerships identified a set of initiatives designed to transform the way health care was delivered by addressing not just the medical needs but also the broader health needs of the local residents. Hospitals played a key role, with a total of sixty-five hospitals represented in the twenty-five CCN partnerships. All subscribed to the four principal goals of the CCN vision:

1. a focus on the health status of communities, not just patients who receive care or enrollees of a health plan;
2. a seamless continuum of care, with mechanisms that facilitate service delivery at the right time in the most appropriate setting;
3. community accountability in terms of identifying collaborative actions based on priority community needs, involving key individuals and organizations in the partnership, and regular reporting of progress to the community; and
4. management within limited resources, the local restructuring of financial resources so that providers are rewarded for keeping people healthy in the most cost-effective way and avoiding duplication of services.

The members of these partnerships include not just health care providers but also public health, schools, businesses, local governments, and social service providers. Through these public–private partnerships, hospitals and other health care organizations are in a better position to address the important social and economic determinants of good health within the communities they serve. Evidence consistently shows that costly, prevalent health care problems stem from "community-level risk factors such as eroding social systems, sociodemographic disparities, violence, sedentary lifestyles, and the aging of the population"[4] If hospitals can work successfully with community-based organizations to address community risk factors, they may be able to positively improve their financial status.[5]

Trustees and managers alike are realizing that no single health services delivery organization can assemble all the resources and capabilities necessary to promote and sustain community/population health. It is dependent on critical factors within a community such as social support, housing, education, and ecology that extend beyond the reach of health service delivery systems. It is in this context that the hospital and its trustees play an important role as citizens in a community.

Thus, it behooves the boards and administrations of health care systems to look outside their doors, beyond the provision of inpatient and ambulatory care, to assess and address the needs of their constituents. By collaborating with other community organizations, hospitals can not only broaden the scope of their efforts and the expertise of those involved but also share the burden of conducting discrete initiatives. For example, one CCN partnership in Cambridge and Somerville, Massachusetts, the Cambridge Health Alliance (CHA), is comprised of two acute care hospitals, a nursing home, the department of public health, a managed care plan, and a network of twenty neighborhood health centers. CHA, in partnership with local schools, ethnic advocacy groups, and civic organizations, is implementing a number of initiatives to improve the quality of life of individuals living in the community.

One such effort is to improve access to culturally appropriate care for rapidly growing immigrant groups in Cambridge and Somerville. To meet the growing need, CHA worked with a local job development agency and a local college focusing on adult education to develop a medical interpreter training program. CHA contributed technical assistance and links to faculty, and, through its two hospital members, helped sell the program to interpreter service directors in other hospitals. In addition to working to expand the pool of trained medical interpreters, CHA worked with an advocacy group to pass legislation that requires Massachusetts hospitals to provide medical interpreters. The business payoff for CHA's investment in improving access to care for immigrant groups was realized in the spring of 2001. At that time, two neighboring hospitals faced closing due, in part, to the fact that their staffing had not kept up with the changing demographic face of their communities. By working with advocacy groups in these communities, CHA paved the path to purchase the two hospi-

tals, and plans are under way to expand the cultural competency of both institutions through the lessons CHA learned in Cambridge and Somerville.[6]

Embedded in this example are some less obvious benefits to health care systems of being involved with their community. Their ongoing community commitment has provided CHA with credibility with state policymakers when
important issues arise. Community residents are willing to go before legislators
and regulatory bodies and endorse CHA proposals because of their positive
expertise.

Satisfaction with a responsive system extends beyond patients. Being mission oriented can help hospitals attract and keep good trustees and employees.
Nurses as well as physicians and trustees are loyal to CHA because they like
their jobs and feel they are making a difference. Most health professionals
choose their careers out of a sincere desire to help others. Where hospitals are
connected to the people they serve, that desire can be fulfilled. And it follows
that employees who are satisfied are less likely to leave, thus decreasing turnover costs and potentially improving continuity of care for patients—which has
the happy result of increasing patient and employee satisfaction.

In addition, especially for systems that include primary care and/or insurance products, preventive, community-based care may be able to decrease
direct costs, even in the short run. Patient-centered appointment systems that
allow for same-day visits allow physicians to see more patients. Access to good,
culturally competent primary care (including prevention, health education, and
screening) can decrease inappropriate and unnecessarily expensive use of the
emergency room. Primary care can improve patients' health, which again adds
to patient and provider satisfaction.

For example, another hospital's engagement in a CCN partnership speaks
directly to the recent Institute of Medicine (IOM) report, *Crossing the Quality
Chasm: A New Health System for the 21st Century,*[7] which challenges hospitals to
"coordinate care across patient conditions, services, and settings over time."
This challenge is clearly linked to the CCN principle of a seamless continuum
of care. As stated in the IOM report, "coordination encompasses a set of practitioner behaviors and information systems intended to bring together health
services, patient needs, and streams of information. It may be facilitated by
procedures for engaging community resources (such as social and public health
services) and other sites of care (such as hospice or home care) when and as
appropriate."

The Decatur Community Partnership, a CCN site in central Illinois, decided
to tackle the problem of patients coming to the hospital's emergency department for nonemergencies. The Decatur Memorial Hospital, the Public Health
Department, and the Community Health Improvement Center (CHIC) began
small, with a pilot program that would allow the partners to test new processes. They targeted a pilot group, CHIC patients, because this group was identi-

fiable, could be reached through the clinic, and had significant needs. Patients enrolled in the program with after-hours needs for medical attention called a central phone number staffed by nurses from the public health department. The nurses followed a standard, computer-generated protocol to determine whether the patient needs to be seen immediately at the emergency room, can wait until the next day for an urgent clinic appointment, can address the problem themselves, or should make a regular clinic appointment for follow-up. The final decision about whether to go to the emergency department was left to the patient, but inappropriate use of the emergency department has decreased by more than 33 percent since the program began.[8]

There are many more examples of how hospital involvement with community partnerships can benefit both the hospital and the broader community it serves. Hospitals that focus on a community-building approach (an approach to sustaining the health of the residents in their communities, not just those in the hospital) should[9]

- engage community members as partners rather than simply as consumers;
- identify existing assets that serve as entry points for community-building activities;
- make strategic investments in existing community assets;
- emphasize community problem solving; and
- make long-term investments in community quality of life.

Returning to the example of the Cambridge Health Alliance, in the late 1990s, administrators and trustees realized that the composition of the Joint Public Health Board (JPHB), which governs CHA's community programming, was not reflective of the communities' ethnic and racial makeup. All members were asked to resign, and a new board—much more diverse—was appointed. Several of the old board members were retained, but others were not. The new chair is a longtime community activist in Somerville. Meetings are now spirited and collegial, with each new board member bringing not only his or her organization's perspective but also personal experiences and knowledge to the table. In the words of Sylvia Saavedra-Keber, executive director of Concilio Hispano and a JPHB member, "as community-based organizations who work with the Latino community, there are just a few of us around who have this type of partnership with the Cambridge Health Alliance, a real partnership. . . . What I mean is not just to refer clients back and forth but to really look at a problem and come and try to resolve that issue together. . . . How is it that we can approach the community together. . . . We can actually get to the policy-makers so we can change the way we conduct and do policy. . . . How is it that we can assist the system in a way to . . . make the system work for the community that it is serving."[10]

Sustaining a Community Health Effort

It is easy enough for a hospital to do a community outreach project or two but much harder to make a serious commitment to community health and to sustain that commitment over years, as populations shift, administrations change, and financial pressures increase. In a recent study of fifteen leading health care organizations, *Sustaining Community Health: The Experience of Health System Leaders*,[11] trustees, administrators, and staff of systems that had won national awards for community health initiatives shared how they had sustained their commitment to community health over time. "Sustainability" is defined here as the ability of health care organizations to move successfully through organizational and business transitions while continuing to meet mission-defined needs, specifically with a focus on improving the health of their communities.

The study suggests that commitments to community health improvement can be sustained even as health care organizations maneuver through difficult dynamics that can dramatically affect their organizational viability. Change was explored in terms of scope of the programs, staffing, and financial resources. While commitments remained intact or grew, the components of the commitments—staffing, programs, dollars, structure—appeared to change in some cases. The study identified likely facilitators and barriers health care organizations encounter when trying to sustain a commitment to community health improvement. Some facilitators can also be barriers. Key facilitators included (1) leadership and board commitment, (2) community partnerships, (3) linkage with the hospital foundation protective structures, and (4) the fiscal health of the organization. Key barriers included (1) the fiscal health of the organization, (2) external funding for community health initiatives, (3) demonstrating a health impact in the community, and (4) demonstrating the value of community health to the organization. Each facilitator and barrier is described below, with case examples.

Leadership and Board Commitment

Visionary leadership at multiple levels within the health care system permeates a commitment throughout the organization that can sustain community health improvement, even in an environment of high chief executive officer turnover. Marian Twombly, director of patient care services at Franklin Regional Hospital in New Hampshire, says, "The hospital must realize that it plays a significant role in the health and social economics of the community; an institution can't be a hospital only." The leadership connection includes the chief executive officer (CEO), board of trustees, and the individual with direct or overall responsibility for community health improvement—usually a vice president or director. The CEO educates the organization and its board of trustees about the importance of community health to the organizational mission, and clarifies its strategic linkage to the organization's clinical and operational areas. In successful community health cultures, the CEO effectively assesses what is needed and provides a clear rationale for how community health fits into the organization's core strategies. The CEO is also often the most visible liaison between the hospital and the rest of the community.

To further this connection, trustees have a particularly important role in recruiting and retaining organizational leadership. Trustees provide a continuity of commitment to community health. During times of transition, it is critical that trustees look for new leadership who will continue that commitment. Trustees also play a critical role in specific strategy approval, budget allocation, and active program participation. For example, trustees sit on the community coalition task forces in Camcare's Kanawha Coalition for Community Health Improvement in Charleston, West Virginia, addressing heart disease prevention, tobacco use reduction, exercise, and dental care. This coalition includes senior leaders from all three local health care organizations as well as the public health department, school system, and other agencies. Trustees sit on community-issue committees at Mount Sinai Hospital Medical Center in Chicago; volunteer in programs established by Franklin Regional Hospital community partners; and mentor students in Oklahoma City Schools for INTEGRIS health. Staff carry out the vision described by the CEO and board of trustees. Leading systems have staff with skills in relating to communities, knowledge of public health, and ability to engage their own organizations financially and programmatically.

COMMUNITY PARTNERSHIPS

Partnerships in the form of community-wide collaborations, issue-specific grassroots coalitions, or shared locations with other community agencies serve to foster the commitment to community health. As Gordon Sprenger from Allina Health Systems (Minneapolis) says, "We have been able to leverage what are limited external dollars in bringing partnerships together. That's what suggested to me that we could sustain community health programs, because it's not all on our back." Camcare's Kanawha Coalition was described as being exceptionally effective in opening the way for organizations to share resources across sectors to solve community health problems.

Another variation of a partnership model is the development of coalitions driven by specific program interests of an individual organization, typically addressing a specific topic. For example, Pitt Partners for Health is a long-standing partnership among University Health Systems of Eastern Carolina (Pitt County Memorial Hospital, Greenville, North Carolina), the University of

Eastern Carolina School of Medicine and School of Health Education, and the local health department. This triad, administratively supported by the health system, is targeting a set of evolving objectives, also based on an extensive household interview and needs assessment. The coalition is also supported by external grants focused on specific areas such as mobile dental services.

Yet another model that works has a health care organization working with an extensive array of partnerships. Parkland Memorial Hospital in Dallas participates in several coalitions, each consisting of as many as dozens of organizations, sometimes including other major health institutions. Each coalition is focused on a specific program area. Examples include the Injury Prevention Center of Greater Dallas, a new Faith–Health Partnership, a coalition effort to Fight Elder Abuse, and a citywide Diabetes Prevention Collaborative.

A different partnership pattern involves co-location of services with different agencies. Mount Sinai's Community Institute rents space to a community-based employment network, a transportation service called Suburban Job Link, and the local Big Brothers and Sisters, all of which represent connections that Mount Sinai has cultivated over several years. Franklin Regional's Caring Community Network of the Twin Rivers culminated in the development of an Intergenerational Community Center offering programs for children, youth, seniors, and welfare recipients.

Trust among the partners, the breadth and extent of the partnerships, and shared decision making are key facilitators to these collaborations. To achieve enduring trust, health care organizations listen to the community to understand their needs and desired outcomes, rather than defining them for the community—not always an easy task. As Lyn Hester of INTEGRIS in Oklahoma City put it, "We thought we knew what communities wanted. We thought the school system needed school nurses and health education. But the school wanted help with medically fragile children, training for their staffing on how to care for them, and they did not want teachers handing out medication. These needs had to be met before there could be a joint perspective on school-based services and access to care initiatives for school-aged children."

PROTECTIVE STRUCTURES

The organizational structure that supports community health improvement can promote the sustainability of the commitment. The leading organizations created distinct departments of community health, foundations, or a 501(c)(3) tax-exempt organization committed to community health. For instance, Mount Sinai contributes operational dollars annually to an independent 501(c)(3), the Sinai Community Institute, part of Sinai Health System. The Sinai Community Institute is directed by a board, which includes trustees, the CEO, and the chief financial officer from Mount Sinai as well as community leaders and members. The hospital continues to support a variety of outreach efforts, such as hospital-based clinical care management projects for chronic diseases like pediatric asthma and two planning task forces devoted to violence and women's health. At the same time, the institute is free to develop its own agenda focusing on health and human services for the local neighborhood and surrounding areas.

Allina has a new Community Investment Advisory Board (CIAB) that evaluates and measures financial and health returns on investment of community health improvement. The CIAB includes the CEO and several members of the board of trustees. The CIAB facilitates the alignment of system-level community health indicators and goals with business-unit community investment planning as part of a decentralized strategic planning process.

Protective structures like these allow for independent agendas, program development, and experimentation separate from the day-to-day operations of the parent organization. They help protect the community health efforts from the budgetary ax when times are tough, perhaps partly by demonstrating the low cost of these efforts compared with the overall organizational budget. Gordon Sprenger of Allina points out: "Community health programming should not be just another line item on a P&L statement. . . . You need to make it tough for the operational folks to see those dollars as a solution to their operational problems."

STRATEGIC ALIGNMENT

The mission statement of most of the leading organizations included a focus on community health. Most organizations also had community health improvement as a corporate objective. True strategic alignment requires buy-in from the operational side of the organization, because community health improvement touches so many operational units. By coordinating resources and activities across units and departments, improving community health becomes not just a goal on paper but a key strategy. Employee awareness of the commitment to community health helps individuals see connections among their efforts, which can lead to leveraging resources and reducing duplication of services. For example, several organizations have realized that some of their existing clinical and marketing programs are actually promoting community health. At INTEGRIS Health, a diabetes screening designed to market the system's clinical services also became an outreach effort to rural communities. Thus staff can begin to look at follow-up numbers, prevalence, access to care, and health status changes. "The goal before might have been to fill doctors' offices," says Lyn Hester. "Now the goal is to prevent or control diabetes."

There are many creative ways to bring community health into alignment with operational goals. Some of these include developing internal communications media, coordinating and facilitating service line involvement, promoting employee involvement, using marketing resources and capitalizing on marketing methods, and cultivating relationships with physicians and other health care professionals. For example, several of the hospitals coordinate an inventory of the community health activities of their business units or departments to coordinate activities, increase visibility, and ensure that all activities are accounted for in community benefit reports. As a result of one such inventory, an organization that thought it had no staff working on community health determined that there were forty-five people working on projects such as community-wide poison-control strategies, epilepsy education, and preventive care.

Of course, the board sets the tone for any strategic alignment. At the Cambridge Health Alliance, the Joint Public Health Board integrates strategic priorities across the hospital, ambulatory system, and board of public health. It also serves as a source of diversity, community-based leadership, and community voice for the entire system.

EVIDENCE OF IMPACT

Evidence that its efforts either improve measurable community health outcomes or decrease institutional costs is a major aid in sustaining a health care organization's commitment to community health improvement. Unfortunately, such evidence is hard to come by; data are not readily available, and it can take a long time to significantly change the health status of a community. Although trustees are justified in seeking data to assess the return on investment from community health initiatives, the complexity and difficulty of providing quick, reliable evidence of their impact must also be realized.

Still, trustees should ask administration and staff to measure success in some meaningful ways based on the purpose of the initiatives. Pitt County Memorial Hospital is using indicators from Healthy People 2010 in the development of their clinical strategic plan. Some leaders report that, in the absence of strong data-based evidence, they have showcased their results by reporting anecdotes and "human" presentations by people who have benefited from the hospital's initiatives. Memorial Health System in South Bend, Indiana, takes its board on an annual Community Plunge to visit program sites and see the community health commitment at work—there is nothing like seeing how a program has helped real people to reinforce people's support for it.

Leading organizations do report that they are beginning to conduct more sophisticated evaluations of their community health activities. At least three sites are building evaluation units to increase their own capability. Parkland

Memorial is starting a Population Medicine Unit and has just completed three surveys in six communities intended to evaluate the impact of their services and current trends. Mount Sinai has established an Urban Health Institute; the Cambridge Health Alliance has started an Institute for Community Health. Allina has also charged its foundation staff with strengthening its approach to evaluation.

Of course, all these efforts require that resources be devoted to evaluation, which is not necessarily an easy sell with staff who are dedicated to "doing the work." But with board leadership, staff can come to see the value of conducting credible evaluations of their work. "Evidence base is most important for the nonbelievers. Most see the common sense of this work, know you have to spend dollars differently, know the time horizons are longer, are tolerant of not having short-term outcome or cost-saving data. There is an appetite for demonstrating short- and long-term results, but you have to be patient," says Tom McBurney of Allina.

Financial Health

Federal and state revenue cutbacks, as well as low managed care payments, are major deterrents to maintaining good financial health and sustaining a commitment to community health. The costs of mergers and acquisitions and failed business ventures have also affected many hospitals' financial ability to support their community health efforts. In some cases, investment income is providing a protective effect. Another way leaders have funded their community health initiatives is by creating a community health investment pool or separate fund. In other cases, growth and increasing market presence have compensated for cuts in reimbursements. Still, many leaders find that it is critical to raise money from external sources—philanthropy; program grants; state vehicles, including tobacco settlement funds and uncompensated care pools; expanded Medicaid managed care programs related to the state children's health insurance programs; and other state health insurance expansions.

In light of public policy that does not provide explicit incentives for a commitment to community health, leaders—namely, trustees and CEOs—must act as advocates for policy change within their communities and their states. "As margins shrink and as the current system of financing your core business continues to be reduced and the resources that you have within your own organization to allocate to those other activities disappear, unless you get some significant changes in the policy of paying institutions for being involved. . . . I don't know where the money is going to come from," explained Phil Goodwin of Camcare. Because private hospitals do not have the same resources or mandate as public hospitals, it is particularly incumbent upon their leaders to advocate for policies that would support a population health approach to community care.

Health care organizations' financial health is the predominant barrier to sustaining a commitment to community health. Each organization needs to evaluate its own situation and focus on strategies that yield the highest return. But first, each organization must answer the fundamental question, "What is truly our role in improving the health of the community?" Once organizations acknowledge their role in improving health status and their responsibility as community-owned facilities, they must embrace community health improvement as a core value and employ strategies to sustain the commitment. Even in the face of turbulent times for health care providers, these fifteen national award-winning organizations and those involved in the twenty-five CCN partnerships have managed to sustain or even strengthen their community health initiatives. With creative thinking, effective implementation tactics, and strong philosophical commitment, the leaders of these hospitals and health systems—CEOs, trustees, and staff—have turned what might seem impossible into practice without ignoring their financial realities. They recognize that in the long run the real question is not "Can we afford to sustain our community health efforts?" but "Can we afford not to?"

NOTES

1. World Health Organization, "Preamble to the Constitution of the World Health Organization as adopted by the International Health Conference," New York, June 19–22, 1946; signed on July 22, 1946, by the representatives of 61 States (*Official Records of the World Health Organization*, no. 2, p. 1) and entered into force on April 7.

2. CNN is the federally registered trademark of First Health Group Corporation for its group health care and workers' compensation preferred provider organization's services. The National Community Care Network Demonstration Program is not affiliated or associated with First Health and its CNN services.

3. The Health Research and Educational Trust, the research and educational affiliate of the American Hospital Association, serves as the national program office for the Community Care Network (CCN) Demonstration Program. For more information or a list of publications about CCN, call the telephone number 312–422–2600.

4. R. G. Evans, M. L. Barer, and T. R. Marmor, eds., *Why Are Some People Healthy and Others Not? The Determinants of Health and of Populations* (New York: Aidene De Gruyter, 1994).

5. B. J. Weiner, J. A. Alexander, and H. S. Zuckerman, "Strategies for Effective Management Participation in Community Health Partnerships," *Health Care Management Review* 25, no. 3 (2000): 48–66.

6. K. Barnett and G. Torres, *Beyond the Medical Model: Hospitals Improve Health through Community Capacity Building*, Community Care Network Issue Brief (Chicago: Health Research and Educational Trust, 2001).

7. Institute of Medicine, *Crossing the Quality Chasm: A New Health System for the 21st Century* (Washington, D.C.: National Academy Press, 2001).

8. M. A. Pittman and F. S. Margolin, "Crossing the Quality Chasm: Steps You Can Take," *Trustee* , July–August 2001.

9. Barnett and Torres, "Beyond the Medical Model."

10. Community Care Networks, *Partnering to Improve Health*, videotape, 2001; available from the Health Research and Educational Trust, Chicago (telephone: 312–422–2600).

11. This section is drawn from the VHA Health Foundation, Inc., and the Health Research and Educational Trust, *Sustaining Community Health: The Experience of Health Care Leaders* (Chicago: Health Research and Educational Trust, 2001). See also Ann Baily, Linda Dewolf, Romana Hasnain Wynia, and Frances Margolin, "Mission Possible: Community Health," *Trustee*, April 2001, 18–22.

5

THE ROLE OF TRUSTEES AND THE ETHICS OF TRUSTEESHIP

Findings from an Empirical Study

Bradford H. Gray and Linda Weiss

Hospitals are vital institutions in most cities and towns, meeting the needs of seriously ill patients, serving as major employers and purchasers, and providing a hub around which countless health and community activities are organized. As nonprofit organizations, most American hospitals are governed by bodies of volunteer citizens, who are commonly chosen for reasons other than expertise in health care administration, disease, or medical care. These trustees have enormous formal responsibility for making crucial strategic decisions and serving as fiduciary in the eyes of regulators. Yet trustees may receive little training, generally have their primary responsibilities elsewhere, and are subject to very little formal oversight.

The institutions for which these trustees are responsible provide crucial technological and caring services to highly vulnerable human beings. Moreover, hospitals are extraordinarily complex institutions. They are capital-intensive organizations that are embedded in a highly competitive market economy with rapidly evolving technologies and great pressure on the bottom line. Nonprofit hospitals are also tax exempt as charitable institutions that receive various forms of public support and are imbued with a great sense of community responsibility. Administratively, hospitals' divisions of labor and lines of authority give them many of the characteristics of bureaucratic organizations. Yet the physicians who make most patient care decisions are generally not even employees of the institution, being in many important respects its *customers*. Moreover, nonprofit hospitals, like their for-profit counterparts, are increasingly part of larger organizational structures in which multiple services are provided through interlocking corporate entities.

Historians teach us that change has always characterized the world of the hospital, but there have been few periods as turbulent as recent years.[1] Two closely related developments have been heavily responsible: (1) new payment methods, particularly Medicare's prospective payment system and the rise of managed care, which have introduced pressures to reduce inpatient care and restrain hospital costs; and (2) outpatient surgery and other changes in the technology of patient care, which have resulted in reduced hospital admissions and shortened lengths of stay. Hospital occupancy has fallen to historical lows—below 60 percent nationally—and thus fixed costs (capital expenses, physical plant, technology) are spread across fewer patients. In addition, the numbers of uninsured Americans has been growing steadily for two decades, reaching 43 million nationally (and, in New York City, 25 percent of the population). All these changes have hit hospitals very hard, because revenues from charges for services constitute the dominant source of operating revenues for most hospitals; few have other significant sources of funds.

Hospitals have adopted many strategies in response to the pressures of the marketplace—offering new services (particularly outpatient services) and seeking ways to combine forces through mergers or strategic alliances. Several hundred nonprofit hospitals have been sold to for-profit purchasers in the past two decades. Several hundred more have closed their doors. Clearly, hospital trustees—whose role once bespoke social position and philanthropy—have been faced with very difficult decisions for which neither they, nor the management teams to which they provide oversight and guidance, have been prepared.

It is in this context that we interviewed hospital trustees and chief executive officers (CEOs) about the role and activities of trustees. Our focus was to examine the moral responsibilities of hospital trustees. The purpose of our interviews was exploratory. We sought to learn more about (1) how trustees define their responsibilities and the extent to which trustees view them in ethical terms, (2) how trustees relate to their hospital and its activities, and (3) the kinds of decisions with which trustees are grappling and the factors that have been pertinent to their decisions. It is intended that our findings will provide some perspective for trustees who are facing significant decisions and provide some insights into changes now occurring in health care delivery and the ways that hospital governing bodies affect those changes.

METHODS

This chapter is based on ninety-eight face-to-face interviews conducted in 1998 and 1999 with trustees and CEOs from two samples of hospitals. The first is a stratified random sample of sixteen hospitals in the greater New York metropolitan area, including Long Island, Westchester County, and the southwestern quadrant of Connecticut. Hospitals were chosen at random from four categories: academic medical centers, other major teaching hospitals, urban community hospitals, and suburban community hospitals.[2] Ten hospitals selected in our original sample declined to participate, and a subsequent sample was drawn. There were additional refusals from urban community hospitals; consequently, that category is underrepresented. The New York–area data, thus, are based on interviews at three academic medical center hospitals, six other teaching hospitals, one urban community hospital, and five suburban community hospitals. For purposes of presentation, we have regrouped these hospitals into just two categories: urban and suburban.

The second sample consists of six hospitals whose trustees had seriously considered either the sale of their institution to a for-profit purchaser or the reorganization of their institution into a for-profit organization. Decisions regarding such matters, we believed, would be among the most difficult that trustees of a nonprofit hospital might face. The hospitals in this "conversion" sample were selected purposively based on several considerations. Most important, we wanted to include hospitals that took the for-profit option and hospitals that did not. We chose four of the former and two of the latter. We wanted recent cases so that memories of trustees' deliberations would be fresh. For practical reasons, we confined ourselves to the eastern United States. Beyond that, we looked for diversity in location and types of institutions, processes used to reach a decision, options considered, and controversy surrounding the decision. We identified cases based primarily on stories in the trade press, supplemented by expert advice. Two of the first six selected refused to participate, and additional selections were made. We ended up with one major teaching hospital, one minor teaching hospital, two suburban hospitals, one urban specialty hospital, and one rehabilitation hospital.

Our research design for both samples called for interviews at each institution with the CEO, board chair, and three other trustees selected by the chair and CEO.[3] We contacted the chair and CEO by letter, requesting their institution's participation, interviews with each of them, and their help in selecting three additional trustees for interviews—one each with particular interest or expertise regarding financial matters, patient care matters, and community concerns. The "finance" trustee chosen for us was typically the chair of the board's finance committee. The "patient care" trustee was generally either the chair of the quality committee or a member of the medical staff who served on the board. The "community" trustees were the most diverse group: Some but not all lived in the neighborhood or community served by the hospital; and some had no apparent tie to the "community" and were probably chosen because of their general knowledge, experience, or commitment to the hospital. Notably, not all the board chairs and members resided in the primary service areas of the hospitals on whose boards they served, although most such individuals worked in some proximity to their hospital.

Because our approach was exploratory, we sought exposure to the range of perspectives that might be brought to the work of trusteeship. The institutions selected and the trustees interviewed did not constitute representative samples in any statistical sense. Our interviews were generally with people who had a strong commitment to the institution and who were among the leaders on their boards.[4] However, the stratified random-sampling procedures used in the selection of institutions and our criteria of diversity of interests in the trustees we interviewed assured that we would be learning about a wide range of circumstances and points of view.

We used a structured interview schedule but digressed to pursue interesting topics. Most of our questions were open-ended. Interviews lasted from forty-five minutes to more than two hours, but averaged about one hour in length. Virtually all were done face-to-face, with two interviewers meeting with the individual being interviewed.[5] Notes were taken during all interviews; most interviews were also tape recorded (with permission) to ensure accuracy and allow for the use of quotations. We were occasionally asked to turn off the tape recorder for discussion of a sensitive issue, and a small number of individuals asked that we not record their interviews. We promised not to identify the institutions or the trustees.

The same procedures were used at the conversion hospitals, but these interviews were somewhat less structured than those in the New York–area sample and, unlike the New York–area interviews, focused heavily on one dominant issue with which the board had grappled. However, on certain key topics, such as how trustees define their responsibilities, we used the same questions in both samples. In reporting our results, we combine responses from the two samples where respondents were asked the same questions.

THE SAMPLE

Some key characteristics of our sample of trustees are presented in table 5.1. Eighty-three percent were male and 89 percent were white. Our interviewees tended toward middle age and retirement years, and many of the trustees had long experience on their boards—several reporting twenty years or more. The

Table 5.1.   Respondent Characteristics by Type of Hospital (*n* = 98[a])

Characteristic	Urban (n = 46)	Suburban (n = 27)	Conversion (n = 25)	Total
Position				
CEO/COO/president	9	6	7	22
Trustee: finance	10	4	5	19
Board chair	10	6	1	17
Trustee: community	8	6	1	15
Trustee: patient care	8	5	2	15
Years on board[b]				
≤ 5	9	6	2	17
> 5, ≤ 10	9	6	9	24
> 10, ≤ 15	3	4	3	10
> 15, ≤ 20	6	1	6	13
> 20	10	4	0	14
Gender				
Female	8	5	3	16
Male	38	22	22	82
Age (years)				
< 40	1	0	0	1
40–49	6	1	0	7
50–59	11	8	2	21
60–69	13	6	0	19
70–79	3	5	1	9
80 +	0	2	0	2
Occupation[b]				
Retired	7	4	3	14
Finance	6	4	4	14
Business	7	3	3	13
Volunteer	3	3	1	7
Health/human services	3	0	3	6
Law	3	3	0	6
Accounting	4	1	0	5
Medicine	0	3	1	4
Academics	1	0	0	1
Ethnicity				
Asian	1	0	0	1
African American	3	1	0	4
Latino	2	0	0	2
White	39	26	23	88
Religion				
Catholic	16	12	7	35
Jewish	16	5	3	24
Protestant	7	6	1	14
Other	1	0	1	2
None	4	2	0	6

Note: CEO = chief executive officer; COO = chief operating officer.
[a] Categories do not all total 98 due to nonresponses and responses that could not be coded.
[b] CEOs not included.

most common occupations of the trustees we interviewed were financial services and business. Some boards included the hospital CEO and some members
of the medical staff; other boards did not. A few individuals without need of
paid work (some were retired and others had sufficient wealth to make a career
out of volunteering) were essentially full-time unpaid trustees. One or two
even had offices in the hospital close to that of the CEO. We encountered such
full-time trustees in five of our hospitals—all of whom were board chairs.

Our sample of trustees included many highly talented, professionally successful, and wealthy individuals. Some had significant business experience, and
many had a sophisticated understanding of trends in the organization and
financing of health care. Others had far less pertinent knowledge or experience.
Within our small group of hospitals, there was obvious diversity across boards
in skills and access to resources, and not all boards had members who would be
considered wealthy or powerful. The academic medical centers had the most
prestigious and best-connected board members, including senior executives of
large corporations, nationally recognized professionals, and persons of great
wealth. We heard examples of such individuals providing major financial support, expert technical advice, and effective advocacy for their institutions
before important funding and regulatory agencies. Smaller urban teaching
hospitals and community hospitals in prosperous suburbs and cities included
professionals (lawyers, accountants, doctors, and financial advisers), business-
persons, and civic leaders, who were generally prominent locally but not
nationally (or not citywide in New York City). Few of these people had the
connections or financial resources found on the boards of the academic medical
centers. The boards of the community hospitals in low-income areas generally
had the fewest resources. Several CEOs described the great difficulties they had
experienced in trying to recruit board members who would bring to the board
pertinent technical knowledge, sophistication about health care, or financial
resources.

The Issues Facing Trustees

Our interviews with CEOs and trustees took place at a time of great turmoil.
Virtually all our institutions had been engaged in issues of enormous importance—facing and contemplating economic collapse, deciding to invest major
resources in the creation of a network with other hospitals, deciding to merge
and give up substantial institutional autonomy, deciding to sell the institution,
or, in one case, deciding to reorganize as a for-profit organization.

Many of the trustees and CEOs we interviewed view this as a uniquely challenging time for hospitals and their trustees, because health care institutions
and providers are "competing for dollars that do not exist," as one CEO put it.

Several mentioned the surplus of hospitals and beds, predicting that some hospitals will eventually close. Some said that the keys to survival might be unknowable. The challenges were described in a number of different ways:

> I would say the primary goal that we have these days is to avoid the red line at the bottom, because times are getting tough. Can we survive? [CEO, suburban community hospital]

> I think this is probably the first time that we've been impacted as much as we have been by the financial situation and that leads to all kinds of struggles. That's probably our most serious challenge, other than building the hospital [in the first place]. [CEO, suburban community hospital]

Many trustees responded in a general way about the difficulties presented by the financing and delivery of health care. Some were more specific regarding the impact of managed care, the serious financial difficulties their hospitals had faced or were currently facing, or the need to change their hospital's services and/or facilities to reflect an increasing emphasis on outpatient care.

We asked our respondents to identify the "two most important issues" with which their board had been engaged in the past year or so. For the institutions that had considered the for-profit conversion item, that issue was clearly dominant. The answers of the respondents in the New York sample are summarized in table 5.2.

The dominant topic for the trustees in our New York sample was decisions regarding affiliations, mergers, or the sale of their institution. Some institutions had recently gone through the process of making such decisions or carrying

Table 5.2.   Topics Identified as One of the "Two Most Important Issues" Dealt with by Hospital Boards in the New York–Area Sample ($n = 16$)

Most Important Issue	No. of Hospitals
Deciding whether the hospital should acquire, merge with, or affiliate with another institution	13
Financial decisions and/or fiscal management	11
Hospital's posture in the turbulent health care environment	7
Enhancing/altering facilities and/or services	6
Physician-related issues	5
Internal management issues	4
Hospital's quality of services	4
Hospital's role in the community	2

Note: We collected this information from each chief executive officer and trustee who we interviewed; because of the consistency among respondents from particular institutions, we present the data with the institution as the unit of analysis.

out such transactions, and they were implementing agreements that had been reached. Others were in the process of forming new relationships with other institutions. Only one institution that had considered options regarding partnering, merging, or sale had drawn back from the decision and decided to remain as a stand-alone institution. Because of the significance of this issue, we have devoted a separate chapter in this volume to it (see chapter 10). Here we will simply summarize these eight issues, pointing in particular to the value dimensions of each. Because they are at the heart of our exploratory approach, these value dimensions are presented in an issue-by-issue fashion in table 5.3. An examination of this table makes it very apparent that there are value components of ethical significance in most major issues dealt with by boards. The eight issues are as follows:

1. *Institutional autonomy.* Thirteen of the boards in our New York–area sample (and all the hospitals in the conversion sample) had considered whether their hospital should merge or affiliate with, or sell to, another hospital or hospital system. These are critically important issues for institutions. Many different arrangements had been considered. In virtually every case, the board had worried about and had tried to assure (1) the hospital's continued presence in the community, (2) the continuation of key aspects of the hospital's mission, or (3) the continuation of the board's voice after the transaction was completed. Virtually no one described his or her board's primary goal in revenue-maximizing terms.

2. *Financial issues.* Respondents from eleven of the institutions in the New York–area sample mentioned financial issues as being among their board's two most important issues in the previous year. Although their phrasing differed, in virtually every case the financial problem pertained to the need to reduce costs. In discussing the factors they had considered, our respondents almost always identified downsides that the board had sought to avoid or minimize— not wanting to lay off staff in their low-income neighborhood, not "becoming the K-Mart of health care," avoiding quality reductions, not closing a clinic on which low-income people depended. As one chair put it, whereas a business can "look at the bottom line of every department and say get rid of everything that loses money, we have to remind ourselves that we have a mission, a Catholic mission, that has to be fulfilled." At the same time, trustees felt responsible for ensuring that the hospital itself remained financially viable.

3. *Positioning the hospital.* In addition to issues involved with mergers and sales, almost half the New York–area sample mentioned that their board had dealt with fundamental issues regarding how the hospital should respond to turbulence in the health care system. This was usually described in rather general terms: "getting our hands around managed care;" responding to competition from the networks of "big city hospitals;" "becoming a significant provider

text continued on p. 112

Table 5.3. The Most Important Issues Dealt with by Boards, Hospital by Hospital, in the New York–Area Sample

Type of Hospital	The "Two Most Important Issues" for the Board, as Identified by Members and Chief Executive Officers (CEOs)	Value Dimensions among the "Most Important Considerations" Regarding These Issues
1. Urban teaching hospital	Whether to affiliate or merge with other institutions to expand patient base.	Described primarily as a business decision. But worry whether the hospital's mission, which emphasizes service, might be threatened if "superstar" doctors are brought in.
		Are benefits of size worth the loss of institutional autonomy?
	How to reduce expenditures in face of budget constraints.	Whether to reduce use of expensive kosher foods. How to avoid compromising care. How to continue to meet responsibilities to serve diverse communities.
	How to prepare for increased federal emphasis on fraud and abuse.	[Issues not described.]
	How to become more flexible and responsive to health system change.	[Issues not described.]
2. Urban community hospital	How to respond to decreasing revenues and remain in business.	Board did not want to lay off people in their impoverished neighborhood.
		To keep money in neighborhood, hospital created fund to enable quick payment of bills to neighborhood businesses.
		Initiated fund-raising campaign.
		Sought help from the state; board members were supportive.

Whether to form an "alliance" with neighboring teaching hospital.	To be sure, issue was "well aired" in the board. Board did not want to give up governance structure; otherwise the decision was easy.
How to shift toward ambulatory care.	[Considerations in decision were not explained by respondent.]
How to increase patient satisfaction ratings.	Decided to aggressively recruit physicians to neighborhood that better matched its ethnic makeup. Required doctors to attend "workshops in sensitivity training" and learn about culture of patients. Took steps to make parking areas safer to be able to recruit better staff.
3. Nonurban community hospital	
Whether to form alliance with another hospital or hospital network.	In addition to business considerations, board wanted to be sure that in joining with a Catholic hospital there would be no "degradation in family planning services," because a section of the community is "dirt poor and desperately need those services."
	Decided not to merge with large network because "we would have been swallowed up," would not have had representatives, and would have lost identity within system.
Whether to build cancer treatment facility with linear accelerator; how to expand services when "ability to raise money was being curtailed."	[Only business considerations mentioned—e.g., how it would be financed. Board did not want to go into debt.]
Physician–hospital integration.	[CEO but no board members mentioned it; issues not described.]

(continues)

Table 5.3.   The Most Important Issues Dealt with by Boards, Hospital by Hospital, in the New York–Area Sample (*Continued*)

Type of Hospital	The "Two Most Important Issues" for the Board, as Identified by Members and Chief Executive Officers (CEOs)	Value Dimensions among the "Most Important Considerations" Regarding These Issues
4. Urban teaching hospital	Becoming part of an integrated delivery system with a top medical school and teaching hospital.	Did not want to "lose ties with the borough" and wanted to maintain services there. Managed to avoid "ceding day-to-day control."
	Confirming ongoing commitment to medical education in the face of funding cuts.	[Issue itself was a value question. They decided to do so.]
	Becoming "involved" with a neighboring hospital that was in trouble.	[Issue itself was a value question, which was debated in business terms—worry about dilution of executive talent.]
5. Urban community hospital	Merger with other hospitals.	Worry about loss of autonomy and how would be represented in governance of combined entity.
		Considered partnering only with other institutions that would maintain Catholic values, including "obligation to the poor," "reproduction, workplace, and economic justice issues."
	Monitoring the "quality and health" of the institution. Dealing with "cash-flow" and "cost-cutting" problems.	Stress on importance of mission, as indicated below.

	How to maintain the care of uninsured patients in the face of "decreased reimbursement from managed care."	"If the hospital survives but has strayed from its mission of caring for people who cannot care for themselves, you haven't accomplished anything." Have sought to address this in the "policy arena" and by being "intimately involved with health care reform efforts."
	Establishing relationship with a tertiary care institution.	Wanted place where tertiary care patients could be sent; also concerns about quality of house staff and integration of medical staffs. Wanted own hospital's doctors to be given proper titles and to be treated "as equals."
6. Nonurban community hospital	How to strengthen the board itself.	Initiative came from management but "board took the bit and ran with it," issues included composition, tasks, and committee structure and responsibilities. Trying to match board member skills and responsibilities.
	How to use Joint Commission on Accreditation of Healthcare Organizations (JCAHO) visit to improve hospital.	Board involved mainly through reports from management.
	Improving relations between community-based and hospital-based physicians.	Worry was that some physicians might take patients elsewhere.
	Worry about increased competition from networks formed by "big city hospitals."	Must respond; "constant reengineering" is part of "good stewardship of the hospital."
	"Managing costs."	Hospital had high mortality rates because of many end-of-life admissions; undertook education program, work with an outpatient hospice program, and are considering starting an inpatient hospice program.

(continues)

Table 5.3. The Most Important Issues Dealt with by Boards, Hospital by Hospital, in the New York–Area Sample (*Continued*)

Type of Hospital	The "Two Most Important Issues" for the Board, as Identified by Members and Chief Executive Officers (CEOs)	Value Dimensions among the "Most Important Considerations" Regarding These Issues
7. Nonurban community hospital	"Finance, which is tied to everything."	"The problem is too many hospitals. Is one going to close? My concern is always, is it us? We were the last one built" [CEO].
		How to prevent other hospitals (in same network) from "stealing" our patients.
	Whether to purchase a $3 million magnetic resonance imaging equipment.	Board recognizes that MDs need proper tools, but believe the expense "would probably bankrupt the hospital, but not buying it would certainly bankrupt the hospital, because doctors would not want to work here. So, we are buying it."
	Growing "conflict between physicians, hospitals, and managed care companies."	"Physicians are very unhappy with managed care. The hospital makes deals that they resent, though we try to be in tandem with the physicians. We recognize they are critical to our operations" [CEO].
	Development of new programs and physical plant.	In past, built center to serve poor women and children. Now considering building an ambulatory surgery center for hospital, because fear losing patients to other hospitals. Question is where to get the money [Trustee 1]. "We are always trying to give community more than what we previously had." In past, built nursing home that is now full, and purchased homes adjacent to hospital for nursing staff when community concerns developed about hospital expanding too close to property line.

8. Urban teaching hospital	Capital formation ("the most important problem in New York City health care is that it is undercapitalized"); immediate issue was building expensive new facility.	Believe patients will be better served with new facility. Idea came from board. Board members have helped raise funds. Board members wanted to be satisfied that need was there.
	Forming joint venture with for-profit firm to offer expensive specialty services.	Board feels competent to deal with "entrepreneurial types" because it has lots of them on it. The board's main concern is better service for the hospital's patients.
	Pursuing the hospital's "commitment to primary, ambulatory care."	Board decided to continue expansion, despite believing that they will lose money "at first." But are also considering closing a center that is losing money. They are struggling with meeting community need, having feeder system for hospital, and operating in financially sound manner.
	Decision against a merger.	Not consistent with their "governing philosophy."
9. Urban teaching hospital	Merger with another major institution for market share, cost control, and reduction in "medical arms race."	"Governance, finance, and organizational structure." Concern about control and its loss. Concern about sustaining the hospital's character as "a personal place." Need to "preserve access." Concern that increased research emphasis might "affect the culture" because different types of physicians will be recruited. Feeling that there were not "cultural" issues between the boards.
	Acquisitions of other hospital to build the network.	Believed will benefit that institution's patients, but there is trustee worry about costs and about whether sufficient information presented to board (rather than to committee).
	The need for budget reductions.	Concerned about impact on quality.

(continues)

Table 5.3. The Most Important Issues Dealt with by Boards, Hospital by Hospital, in the New York–Area Sample *(Continued)*

Type of Hospital	The "Two Most Important Issues" for the Board, as Identified by Members and Chief Executive Officers (CEOs)	Value Dimensions among the "Most Important Considerations" Regarding These Issues
10. Urban community hospital	"Affiliation" with hospital in neighboring community.	Will add "political clout" needed for survival of the hospital. Some board members had "ego problems" with losing power. Decided against merging with large hospital for fear that it would not be concerned with their problems; merged instead with similarly sized hospital in neighboring community.
	Physician "contentment" and satisfaction.	Physicians being hurt by managed care want salaried positions in hospital, but positions are not available. Try to appeal by improving aesthetics, responsiveness of admitting office, and quality of nursing staff. Having several physicians on board is thought to be helpful.
		Chief operating officer sees ethical problems in meeting demands of doctors who are taking their patients elsewhere; some who would admit are "probably OK but not great." How do we attract back the doctors who have shifted admitting patterns while, because of the hospital's financial distress, stronger internal controls are needed? Worry about having to "give them things that make them want to practice here" while having to lay off low-level staff who really need jobs.
	Money. How to bring in more and spend less. Hospital verged on bankruptcy, prevented only by a state bailout. Affiliation was the result.	Considering reducing the residency program to get more money under the Health Care Financing Administration program. Looking for ways to do more outreach and ambulatory care (as business decision to bring in money).

11. Nonurban community hospital

Reorganization, changing administration, and cleaning up problems from previous management, who thought of the hospital in "one-on-one patient care terms" rather than "globally." ("changing from mom-and-pop store to supermarket"). Medical records and accounts payable had been disasters.

Board set up "watchdog committee" to make sure "problems are cleaned up in timely fashion." The board "now realizes that the hospital must be run like a business." Now have finance officer who responds to finance committee requests and prepares reports. (Previous finance officer embezzled hospital funds.) Hope new management and the affiliation will result in all of these problems being addressed.

Affiliation (not merger) with larger hospital, which is seen as necessary because the hospital's previous isolation from managed care is quickly ending.

Wanted to maintain quality and autonomy of hospital. Looking not for "salvation" but for strengthening; want people in community to continue to see the doctor they've been seeing and to use the hospital that they have been using. "Independence is revered here," but "if all other hospitals have aggregated into larger systems, you can be out of business because all the contracts will have gone to them" [CEO].

MD board member: "The process [reaffiliation] has had very heavy physician involvement. ... Doctors' view is key; if the doctors do not buy in, it will not work.

Reducing costs. Also described as "how to deliver health care in today's environment."

Goal to make hospital competitive without becoming "K-Mart of health care." Alternative to cost containment described as bankruptcy, though hospital is in the black and has little debt.

Need "to reduce costs and downsize without losing mission and capability."

(continues)

Table 5.3. The Most Important Issues Dealt with by Boards, Hospital by Hospital, in the New York–Area Sample (*Continued*)

Type of Hospital	The "Two Most Important Issues" for the Board, as Identified by Members and Chief Executive Officers (CEOs)	Value Dimensions among the "Most Important Considerations" Regarding These Issues
	How to "bring together all the diverse interests—doctors, communities, and the board—so that they all work together."	Board gets information not only from management but also from their other roles in the community.
	Meeting community needs while facing financial realities.	Trustee: "In old days, the hospital was the center of the health care delivery system. Now as a facility it is less and less important and one has to look outside its walls. . . . Needs are now teen pregnancy, poor elderly. The hospital has to meet those needs even though they don't make money." As result of this logic, the hospital built nursing home and community health center in recent years.
12. Urban teaching hospital	Fund-raising for new facility.	The board played major role in this.
	Merging with another major hospital and building network of facilities.	Wanted "suitable partner" [that was] "their equal."
		Board had concerns about debt and about "what will happen to board members" when merger occurs. Leaders sought to avoid "offending" or "pushing out" talented people from both board and management.

		Concerns about implications for institutions' teaching activities.
		Major concern was increasing quality of care via the merger, not downsizing for efficiency sake, though "financial advantages" were expected.
		A board committee is playing a role in "helping people understand what the merged institution is."
13. Urban teaching hospital	Merger with another major hospital.	Chair: "For all, the motivation is the pursuit of world excellence." Most decisions were business decisions re management of combined entities, reconciling the institutions' differing premerger strategies, and getting key parties on board.
		Member: felt merger was best way to meet "need to provide outstanding research and world-class clinical care." Members wanted to be sure that mission as relates to community would not be affected and that CEOs and boards would "get along." Was seen as "merger of equals" of institutions that had "complementary" strengths.
	Getting institution back to "full strength" and "solidifying the management group."	No board role described. "Survival was the strong motivating consideration."
	To fill some key clinical positions.	No board role was described, though the issue was identified by a board member.

(continues)

Table 5.3.   The Most Important Issues Dealt with by Boards, Hospital by Hospital, in the New York–Area Sample (*Continued*)

Type of Hospital	The "Two Most Important Issues" for the Board, as Identified by Members and Chief Executive Officers (CEOs)	Value Dimensions among the "Most Important Considerations" Regarding These Issues
14. Urban community hospital	Creating affiliation relationship with academic medical center, once convinced that hospital could not stand alone. Received financial assistance in the "sponsorship" deal that was struck.	CEO describes it as "a business issue." Board wanted to remain a community hospital, not just serve as ambulatory feeder for a larger hospital; this shaped choice of partner. Board member: "In the euphoria resulting from receiving financial assistance, it would be easy to lose sight of the Faustian transaction taking place. I personally made sure that every board member was reminded at every meeting that they were permanently giving up their independence. . . . Trustees must be sure that changing the structure in this way serves their purpose." Board had to recognize that the hospital was becoming a "wholly owned subsidiary" and that the sponsoring organization could "replace the full board at a whim." They believe that current leadership of sponsoring organization shares commitment to the community; the worry that when different leadership comes in, it might feel different. Board member: my concern was to ensure that the hospital would still be able to serve the population of this community.

Issues pertaining to quality and board's meaningful involvement with it.	In preparation for JCAHO, reorganized quality assurance activities in hospital and sought to produce information that the board can digest and use to provide input.
Getting "hands around the managed care issue" and setting up physician health network and "single signature" contracting ability for hospital and medical staff.	Board wanted to be sure the hospital could "retain and recruit qualified physicians who would align with the institution as partners."
Changing CEOs.	Doctors resisted change: "It has been a learning experience for trustees, administrators, and doctors."
	Board formed small group. Defined qualifications desired and then loosened them "when we realized what we could afford to pay." Wanted strong operating skills.
Building market share.	Opening satellites and having presence in more neighborhoods.
Financial implications of changing information technology because required big investment.	[Business decision dealt with by strategic planning and finance committees of board.] Doing it in stages because lack funds to do at once, which would be cheaper.
15. Urban community hospital	
Finance and cash flow problems and need to cut costs. Seen by CEO and board as result of payer policies re slow payments, inadequate rates, coverage denials for the emergency room. "At the mercy of funders."	Chair: A board with "active successful executives" tends to think of the hospital in same way as any other business, to "look at bottom line of every department and say get rid of everything that loses money. We have to remind ourselves that they have a mission—a Catholic mission—that has to be fulfilled." Their mission requires keeping money-losing neonatal intensive care unit open "because we are supposed to take care of children that are orphaned and unwed mothers and their children." Like a supermarket may lose money on 800 products but make it up on 200, a hospital must "look for services that make money to allow for continuation of services that help fulfill mission."

(continues)

Table 5.3.   The Most Important Issues Dealt with by Boards, Hospital by Hospital, in the New York–Area Sample *(Continued)*

Type of Hospital	The "Two Most Important Issues" for the Board, as Identified by Members and Chief Executive Officers (CEOs)	Value Dimensions among the "Most Important Considerations" Regarding These Issues
	How to position hospital to move forward with the vision of becoming a "significant provider of health care in the Northeast U.S."	Member: Undertaking "extremely risky" new activities that involved attracting very prominent specialists from other institutions. Have had to build expensive new specialized facility for this, while they "are struggling to survive."
	Struggling with expansion versus steady state versus cutting back. Which to do?	Member: The board and CEO "are engaged in what is probably the most complex work in our society . . . involving welfare, well-being, the health of society, values in society. . . . Everything is transforming. I've never seen such complicated work. I didn't realize it would be like that. I keep trying to learn and to be very careful." To make decisions, we "must consider our core mission and the core values of the institution. What do we believe in? What should we be doing? We must hold onto certain things, like not jeopardizing quality patient care. We never purposely reduce the care provided. We would give up research before giving up patient care. . . . A hospital is not a corporation. It is about human beings, which makes things more complicated."

16. Nonurban community hospital	Finances for upgrading and modernizing facility.	Board cut back plan drastically to make sure that "we would be able to pay back the money borrowed." "At first we cut rationally, but it eventually got to the point where we had to go beyond the rational." Also board needed to assure that clinical facilities upgraded were consistent with strategic plan regarding "the need to switch our focus to outpatient care."
	Affiliation with local hospital network; survival required it.	Described as business decision to "counteract the HMOs [health maintenance organizations]." Chose what one member said was stronger of the two affiliation alternatives; another said chose on basis of best fits of missions. Also, "retaining community control and identity had to be translated into the actual sponsorship agreement." In the rejected alternative, board members feared their hospital, which was the smaller and weaker institution, would have been "raped" and then closed down.
	Renegotiating labor contract.	"Not a board issue . . . but board has gotten involved [by] volunteering to fill in for striking workers. We'll even clean the toilets."

Note: The terminology used is almost all in the words of the respondents but has been compressed for ease of presentation.

in the Northeast U.S.;" shifting toward ambulatory care; becoming more flexible and responsive to health system change.

4. *Facility enhancement.* For 30 percent of the institutions in our New York–area sample, questions about enhancing or altering facilities had been major board issues in the previous year. The considerations involved pertained to enhancing quality, meeting unmet needs, and accessing needed capital. These decisions could be very difficult on business grounds alone. For example, a trustee at a financially struggling institution described the options underlying the board's decision to spend several million dollars on a magnetic resonance imaging system. The expense "would *probably* bankrupt the hospital, but not buying it would *certainly* bankrupt the hospital, because doctors would not want to work here. So, we are buying it." But most of the trustees also mentioned issues that fell outside the economic calculus, including various aspects of the hospital's service mission.

5. *Physician relations.* Several respondents indicated that issues pertaining to the hospital's relationships with physicians had been important for their board. Physician-related issues mentioned here (and in response to other questions) included recruitment, responding to physician-related quality problems, deciding whether proposed investments would benefit primarily the doctors rather than the hospital, making trade-offs regarding expenditures versus the risk that doctors would take patients elsewhere, and arguing about fairness in hospital–physician joint ventures.

6. *Managerial issues.* Respondents from one-fourth of the hospitals indicated that matters pertaining to governance and management had been among their board's most important issues. Topics mentioned included reorganizing and strengthening the management team, improving the board itself (either its skills or composition), setting up a board "watchdog committee" to oversee management, and keeping the hospital functioning during a labor dispute.

7. *Quality of services.* At most institutions, certain board members had responsibilities related to quality, such as service on the hospital quality-improvement committee. Beyond that, respondents from a handful of hospitals mentioned quality as among the major issues for the board in the previous year. These issues were often described in vague terms (e.g., "monitoring quality"), but several concrete problems were mentioned, such as using a visit from a Joint Commission on Accreditation of Healthcare Organizations to improve quality, seek ways to improve patient satisfaction, and get the board more meaningfully involved with quality.

8. *Community role.* Particular concerns mentioned here included deciding whether and how to help a neighboring hospital that was in trouble; considering "how to bring together all the diverse interests—doctors, communities, and the board—to work together" to meet community needs; how to deliver health care services outside the hospital building, particularly when those ser-

vices do not make money; and caring for increasing numbers of uninsured patients.

How Trustees View Their Responsibilities

Early in our interviews, before any discussion of the issues with which they had been engaged, we asked trustees and CEOs to describe their view of "the responsibility of trustees at this institution." This question was asked in an open-ended fashion, without our suggesting categories into which trustees might fit their responses. Trustees were not asked to prioritize their answers. Most respondents mentioned several responsibilities. The way that answers were formulated was highly varied, and many had explicit or implicit ethical overtones. We grouped the responses according to several themes—oversight, policymaking, the board–CEO relationship, the hospital's charitable role, representational issues, fund-raising and advocacy, and proper behaviors for trustees.

The Oversight Role

Ninety-one of the ninety-eight trustees and CEOs we interviewed defined board members' responsibilities in terms of oversight. The ways they described their oversight responsibilities were quite variable, however. Some trustees stated their oversight responsibilities in operational terms, focusing on the day-to-day work of the hospital (e.g., to be sure that the hospital is providing good patient care), while others used more conceptual terms (e.g., to engage in planning and goal setting).

The oversight responsibility was framed in quite diverse ways, and many respondents mentioned several forms or aspects of oversight. Forty-three respondents referred to *financial* oversight of the institution, most commonly stated in terms of "fiduciary responsibility," assuring the financial soundness of the institution, or simply "stewardship." Thirty-six respondents referred to the *community*, often again using the language of fiduciary responsibility. The following quotes come from five different institutions:

> Trustees have a fiduciary responsibility to make sure that resources given to the hospital are used properly. We represent the community in assuming this responsibility. [Trustee, urban hospital]

> We hold the hospital in trust for the community. [Chair, community hospital]

> We have a responsibility to the community to maintain the hospital so that it can effectively meet the needs of the community. If the hospital isn't strong, then it's not doing its job for the community. [Chair, urban hospital]

Their responsibility is to protect and assure the survival and viability of the institution. If this is a community resource, their responsibility is to protect, preserve, and hopefully improve it. [CEO, major teaching hospital]

Trustees have to ensure that the hospital is appropriately sized and staffed to meet the needs of [the communities it serves], to ensure that there is an environment in which physicians can thrive, and that there is quality and appropriate care and programs for patients. [Trustee, major teaching hospital]

Thirty-two respondents mentioned quality of care as a trustee responsibility, with some noting that this is a legal responsibility of trustees in New York. Twenty-eight respondents defined trustees' responsibilities in terms of the hospital's mission, using language such as the following:

[Trustees are] to support and uphold the mission of the institution—to make sure we are following what the mission is and doing it in a way that is financially responsible. [CEO, teaching hospital]

. . . to ensure that the mission is carried out in a compassionate manner. [Trustee, teaching hospital]

. . . to develop and ratify the mission for the institution and to oversee the fulfillment of the mission. [CEO, community hospital]

Trustees must believe in the mission and have a part in the oversight and implementation of the mission. They support the CEO and staff in various ways, like asking questions, making suggestions, lending expertise. [Trustee, community hospital]

Ten respondents said that trustees' responsibilities included seeing that the hospital followed its *policies* or achieved its *goals*. Eight mentioned having *legal* responsibility. Twenty respondents simply said that trustees are responsible for oversight in general or for "everything," as in the following:

Well of course, ultimately [we're] responsible for everything that happens at the institution. As a practical matter, the [trustee's] primary responsibility is to ensure that to the best of his ability—his or her ability—that the systems and procedures are in place to ensure that the care delivered is of the highest quality and that it is delivered in a financially responsible manner. And much flows from that. [Chair, teaching hospital]

In a similar vein, two respondents described the trustee's role in terms of serving as the "safety-net" for the institution. More apocalyptically, seven respondents defined the trustee's role as assuring the survival of their institution.[6]

The vocabulary of *ethics* came up only three times in trustees' discussions of their responsibilities, all in the oversight context. The formulations were that trustees should "ensure that the hospital provides ethical and appropriate services" [chair, urban hospital]; that trustees should "make sure the hospital is fiscally and socially responsible" [trustee, major teaching hospital]; and that trustees are responsible for "ensuring that the hospital is run in an ethical and financially secure manner" [member, urban community hospital]. Of course, many other trustee comments in response to this and other questions show that trustees are engaged with ethical issues, even if they do not use the vocabulary of ethics to define their responsibilities.

The Policymaking Role

Because almost all respondents included *oversight* in their conception of the responsibilities of trustees, it is notable that few mentioned *policymaking* as a responsibility of trustees. Sixteen respondents indicated that a trustee's responsibilities include setting *institutional goals or policies*, but only two said that their responsibility included defining or setting the institution's *mission*. (Recall that twenty-three respondents had said that a trustee's responsibilities include oversight of whether the hospital is *adhering to* its mission.) Several other responses arguably pertained to policymaking. Thus, six respondents who did not refer to policymaking mentioned responsibility to make resource allocation decisions or to deal with economic constraints, and twelve referred to a trustee role in strategic planning. Four trustees said that their job included setting important aspects of the institutional culture—that the institution be run with compassion, that it engage in the pursuit of excellence, and that it be run for the benefit of patients.

The Board–CEO Relationship

In describing trustees' responsibilities, forty-five respondents (thirty-two trustees and thirteen CEOs) mentioned the hospital's *management*—more than mentioned the community and its needs (thirty-six), the hospital's mission (twenty-eight), patients (nine), or doctors and nurses (one). As has already been noted, *oversight of* management was a common response, mentioned by thirty-two respondents (including eleven of the twenty-one CEOs who were interviewed). But management was mentioned in several other ways. Thus, twelve respondents mentioned the hiring and firing of CEOs as a trustee responsibility, and ten suggested that a trustee's responsibilities included "supporting" or serving as a sounding board for management.

Sixteen of the respondents who defined a trustee's responsibilities in terms of oversight of management went on to distinguish how the trustee's role differs from the role of management, as in the following:

[The board's job] is to select the CEO and monitor his performance, to ratify his decisions, change his mind, or replace him. If too much is done by trustees regarding running the organization, it brings mediocrity. [Trustee, urban teaching hospital]

[The trustee's job] is to see that the CEO and administration perform according to the mission and bylaws of the institution. [Chair, urban hospital]

We're not running the hospital. We're setting the broad policy under which people that we chose are running the hospital. If we get unhappy with the way the hospital is run, then we get a new CEO. [Chair, teaching hospital]

The Hospital as a Charitable Institution

In contrast to those who framed trustees' responsibilities in the relatively abstract terms of community needs, missions, goals, and oversight of management, a handful of respondents (seven) defined trustees' responsibilities in terms of charitable activities or the ways that decisions appropriate to their hospital might differ from decisions made regarding a business. Here are some examples of these statements:

[The trustee's responsibility is] to make sure that the hospital does not stray from its mission because of economics, [even though] serving the community is hard with the economic constraints that we face. [Chair, suburban hospital]

I think one of the conflicts you get into occasionally is you've got to run a business, but you've got to take care of people and [consider] how do you do that effectively. You can't lose sight of the fact that you're here really to take care of people, but if you don't keep your financial situation strong, you're not going to be there to do the job. [Trustee, community hospital]

[The trustee should] support and uphold the mission of the institution, including activities that don't enhance the bottom line. [Trustee, urban teaching hospital]

[The trustee should] make sure that the hospital does not stray from mission because of economics. [Chair, urban hospital]

To make sure that care is available without regard to ability to pay. [Trustee, urban hospital]

To balance financial fiduciary responsibility against community need—including services that lose money. It is different than a for-profit. [Trustee, hospital that decided against sale to a for-profit company]

The bottom line keeps for-profits disciplined. Trustees should want to "run a tight ship," but the hospital should cover some uncompensated care. [Trustee, hospital that had decided to reorganize as a for-profit]

The infrequent mention of the hospital's charitable behavior in descriptions of the role of trustees appears not to be an accurate reflection of hospitals' policies. In response to a later question regarding whether their board had discussed charity care in the past year, trustees from virtually every institution replied affirmatively and then volunteered that the hospital's policies are to provide care without regard to ability to pay. Moreover, in describing issues with which their boards had grappled during the past year, decisions affecting charity care came up several times (e.g., whether to invest in a health center in an underserved, poor neighborhood; and whether to close a clinic that served poor people because of the magnitude of financial losses). Still, charity care does not seem to be at the forefront of trustees' and CEOs' thinking when defining the responsibilities of trustees, although this may have been implicit in their thinking when they mentioned responsiveness to community needs or seeing that the hospital pursues its mission.

Issues Regarding Representation

An important issue regarding hospital governance is whether it is a trustee's job to exercise independent judgment versus being there to represent a constituency. In responding to our question about the responsibility of trustees, only six respondents said that trustees serve as *representatives*. The categories they saw themselves as representing were very broad: the hospital's "constituencies," " the community or communities served by the hospital," the "people of New York," or "the population who uses the hospital." Although one might imagine that trustees who see themselves as representatives might be drawn from relatively small communities, five of these six respondents were from hospitals in New York City (with three from major teaching institutions).

After asking our question about the responsibilities of trustees, we directly asked trustees whether they viewed themselves as "representing any particular interest or group." Most (thirty-eight) said that they did not, and eighteen said that they represent the community or the "public at large." Seven trustees said that they represent the hospital itself (including doctors and patients), and four said they represent patients (including one who said he represented both physicians and patients). Two said they represented uninsured and poor people. The chair of a Catholic hospital said that he represents the diocese "to ensure that the hospital is faithful to the church and the church's mission to serve the disadvantaged." A businessman in a small Connecticut city responded frankly when asked if he represented any particular interest or group: "Not really, but I'm a member of the community and my company is here. It is one of the largest employers in the area and my employees use the hospital." One trustee described herself as "pro-nurse," observing that men on the board "wanted to cut the nursing staff, but I always try to preserve it. I fight as hard as I can for them."

The presence of physicians on boards elicited comment. One trustee, who was also his hospital's medical director, observed that the trustee's first interest is the community but that as medical director, "I have to be a proponent for the employees and the medical staff." A trustee from another institution said that he had favored physician involvement in the board, but he said that their role was "not to represent physicians—they [like everyone else] were there to represent the community." A physician/board member defended the physician's role on boards, saying, "I represent the clinical reality of patient care. The board is the fiduciary for the financial side of the hospital and is dominated by people with that concern. So, clinical input is important."

Several trustees' comments suggested strong reservations about the idea of trustee as representative. One reservation concerned not wanting to be viewed by other trustees in such terms. Thus, one woman said that when she joined the board, she had made sure that she would not be "pigeonholed into women's issues"; a chairperson of an urban hospital said, "I would like to think that people see me as more than Puerto Rican"; and a trustee said that as the only black person on her board, "people might think that I represent the black community, but I don't see myself that way." Another African American woman said that she did not see herself as representing any particular group and, furthermore, "I'm not expected to do so, and that is a good thing." A second reservation pertained to the appropriate view of the responsibility of trustees: In explaining his saying that he does not represent any particular interest or group, one trustee said that "board members have to understand that the output is health care. If your objective is something different, you shouldn't be on the board." A chairman combined both of these points: "You want to have a wide spectrum of people on your board, but you don't want to put on them the burden of trying to represent something. What they represent is their judgment. If it's a black member of the board, he's had a 'black experience' and brings that sensitivity."

A trustee at another institution linked the idea of representation with a concern about qualifications. He said that he does not represent any interest or group and was "against the idea in general." He said that their board's one African American, who holds a responsible professional position in the community, "advocates for more minority representation," but our respondent stated that the board "should not take someone for whom they represent—they must have the proper qualifications and be willing to spend the time needed." He expressed concern that a board made up of people serving in a representational capacity would result in the hospitals' having "little fiefdoms." He said that he had argued with his African American colleague about this issue.

The complexities that this question elicited for some members of minority groups were well stated by a Puerto Rican woman who serves on the board of a major teaching institution. Asked if she represented any particular interest or group, she observed, "I represent people who like change, who like action, and who are against the status quo." She said that she also brings the perspective of a working woman, observing that the only women on the board when she came on "were wives of." Because she is Puerto Rican, she noted, she can tell the board when they are doing something that is "elitist," and she can give the hospital entry into a large and important minority community. And a Chinese board member at an urban hospital characterized herself as representing "the patient population," which she then noted was 50 percent Chinese.

A few members expressed approval of the representation model of trusteeship. A well-known attorney who is a trustee of a New York hospital told us that although he, himself, did not represent any interest or group, some others on the board "represent different groups, like important community institutions." This was said without a hint of disapproval. And even some who claimed to be advocates for a particular interest did so in ways that conveyed some uncertainty about whether that was appropriate. A trustee (not the one quoted above regarding nursing) told us that she has a particular area in nursing and watches developments there closely; but she then said that she is not a "special advocate" for nurses, because "that would not be appropriate." She then stated that she is "an advocate of the administration, a strong patient advocate, and an advocate of the public trust."

Financial and Other Forms of Support

Responses to our question about "the responsibility of trustees at this hospital" elicited several responses that go beyond the governance role. Five respondents said that trustees should serve as advocates *for* the institution in community, regulatory, and policymaking contexts. Eight respondents (four trustees and four CEOs) mentioned the philanthropic or fund-raising role of trustees, but not necessarily in an expected way. Only seven described fund-raising as part of the responsibilities of trustees, with one CEO describing it as helping the hospital "go beyond what is practical," one trustee describing it as "giving and getting," and one CEO lamenting that his board did not do enough of it. One respondent characterized the trustee's fund-raising role as something that was part of the past. Whether or not that is true, fewer than 10 percent of our respondents mentioned it when they were asked about trustees' responsibilities.

However, elsewhere in our interviews many trustees mentioned significant financial contributions that they or their fellow trustees had made to their institution. A CEO whose hospital had just announced a large capital campaign for a new facility told us with great pride of the millions of dollars that members of his board had contributed to launch the campaign. At many institutions we visited, evidence of past contributions by board members could be seen either in the names of buildings and wings or on plaques adorning the walls. Despite such recognition given for large contributions, many CEOs and trustees interviewed seemed to view their philanthropic contributions as voluntary acts done out of admiration of the institution, not as an obligation of trusteeship. Or perhaps giving money is expected only from some trustees and is not seen as an obligation that applies to trustees generally. Several CEOs and trustees lamented that their hospital had not been able to recruit trustees who have the ability to make ample contributions. Some felt that trustees did not do everything that they could in this regard, as with the board chair of a teaching hospital that serves primarily low-income communities who observed sadly that members of his board "haven't supplied the voluntary contributions that could make a difference."

The Behavior of Trustees

Some trustees responded to our question about the responsibilities of trustees not by discussing the substantive matters with which trustees should be concerned but, instead, by discussing how they should carry out their role. Thus, eight respondents referred to the way that trustees should approach the job—be diligent, interested, or committed; not be self-interested; or use good judgment or bring expertise. Ten respondents discussed trustees' responsibilities in terms of how trustees should behave, using phrases such as "ask questions and get answers," "learn what's going on," and "keep up with the changing environment."

In terms of how trustees actually carry out their responsibilities, there is also significant variability. On the one hand, we were told in a few institutions of trustees who just attend meetings in which little goes on. This was sometimes blamed on the trustees themselves and their lack of interest or lack of skills. A small number questioned whether it is possible for trustees to play a meaningful role in the governance of the modern hospital. As the CEO of a community hospital described, with some bitterness:

> In today's corporate world boards are less and less meaningful in terms of operations. The damn thing's become so complicated it's impossible to explain. . . . So, the practical answer is I need them for their money, I need them for their name, and I guess for a major decision—should we go to war with China?—yes, alright I need them for that. But all the rest, I can do it myself, and *do* do it myself, and *have to* do it myself. When I'm short and can't meet payroll, they're not at home. I sweat at night and I wonder and I wake up at 2 o'clock in the morning and say, "what the hell am I going to do next?"

On the other hand, we also interviewed trustees who are deeply involved with their hospital on a daily basis, with significant positive impact on their institutions. This was particularly true during periods of crisis or when major decisions were being made (like a sale or partnering arrangement with another institution). But for some trustees, it was simply how they approached their job. We met trustees who walk the floors of their hospital regularly, who answer mail from disgruntled (or satisfied) staff and patients, who provide advice to patients on a choice of physicians (or who make referrals thereto), or who take on significant administrative responsibilities. Twenty-three percent of the trustees we interviewed told us that they spent more than ten hours a week on board- and hospital-related work, and seven people (all board chairs) said that they devoted more than twenty hours a week to the hospital.

Observations about How Trustees' Responsibilities Are Viewed

The responses to our question about the responsibilities of trustees at their institution produced a wide range of responses. Two points are worthy of emphasis. First, few of the differences in conceptions of a trustee's responsibility appear to be mutually incompatible. Rather, they are differences in emphasis. Second, the importance of diversity within boards becomes clear in these responses, to guard against the imbalances that might result from an exclusive concern with certain dimensions (e.g., financial soundness) at the expense of other priorities (e.g., meeting important community needs).

Also notable is the fact that trustees described their responsibilities much more commonly in terms of various forms and aspects of oversight of hospital operations than in terms of a forward-looking, strategic planning role. What is interesting about this, as was noted above, is that many of the institutions we visited had been engaged in decision making regarding the very future of their institution as an independent entity. Even so, the conceptions of their responsibilities that we heard from our respondents put much more emphasis on ongoing oversight than on planning for the future. Perhaps this is a measure of trustees' lack of preparedness for the types of decisions that they faced in the late 1990s.

Finally, although a presentation of variations among trustees and institutions is beyond the scope of this chapter, it is clear that such differences exist. We noticed, for example, that CEOs were much more likely than trustees to identify oversight of the CEO as a trustee responsibility. Trustees were much more likely than CEOs to define their responsibility as assuring that community needs were met. Trustees and CEOs at hospitals that had considered the for-profit sale of their institution were the most likely to identify the definition of mission as a responsibility of trustees. The trustees of urban hospitals had a much greater focus than suburban trustees on oversight of the fiscal and operational aspects of their hospital, while trustees at suburban hospitals were more likely than urban trustees to identify meeting community needs as a trustee responsibility. Trustees of community hospitals, hospitals with a religious affiliation, and hospitals located in low-income areas were particularly likely to define their responsibilities in terms of the surrounding community and/or low-income or otherwise disadvantaged populations.

Trustees' Definitions of Ethics

To learn how trustees themselves view the ethical dimensions of their role, we asked the following question: "Of the issues that the board has considered over the last few years, are there any that you think of as ethical issues?" This question was asked early in the interview, before any other question regarding issues with which the board had been engaged.[7] It was apparent most trustees and CEOs had not thought before of such a question, and the typical initial response was a long pause for thought about it.

However, only eight respondents told us that their board had dealt with no ethical issues at all. (One, taking the question to refer to the issue of abortion, said that it would be inappropriate for trustees to bring their views of the matter into the boardroom.) The remaining eighty-one respondents identified ethical issues—though not always in terms of issues that had arisen in the past year and not always in terms of matters that had involved an actual board decision (as opposed to being briefed on the topic).

Some of the issues defined as "ethical" pertained to what we term the ethics *of* trusteeship—involving the composition of the board or the behavior of board members themselves. Most of the issues about which we were told pertained to ethics *in* trusteeship—substantive matters about which boards had made decisions or been briefed. In view of the purpose of this chapter, we will attempt to convey the nature of the full range of these concerns.

Ethics of Trusteeship

For fifteen of our respondents, the question about ethical issues dealt with by the board produced responses regarding either conflict of interest or board composition. For thirteen respondents, our question brought to mind conflict-of-interest situations involving trustees who form decisions that the board makes. Six respondents (from five institutions—one-fourth of the total) said that they had current or recent conflict-of-interest problems on their board. Two of these cases involved physicians, and related to decisions that might affect their incomes. The other instances involved trustees who were thought to have benefited from doing business with the hospital.

In two instances, both of which were from hospitals that had considered sale of the institution, trustee conflicts of interest had created crises in the past. In one instance, a public scandal had developed that had discredited the hospital. In the other instance, a group of medical staff members who objected to a board decision regarding the sale of the institution compiled a dossier of supposed conflicts of interest of board members (and their families) who had allegedly done business (banking, construction, architecture) with the hospital. They threatened to take out a newspaper advertisement accusing board members of profiteering. Although the trustees whom we interviewed raised questions about the fairness or validity of the conflict-of-interest allegations, the threat led to the resignation of most members of the board and effectively blocked the decision to sell the hospital. Clearly, the perception that trustees who are making important decisions have used their position to gain private benefit can have an enormous negative impact on a board's ability to function.

A different conflict-of-interest issue was described at an institution that had been created by the merger of two formerly competing hospitals in neighboring communities. As the CEO described it:

> There are always personal ethics in board member conduct. Many board members have allegiances. They have to face the fact that their allegiance must be to the community as a whole, not to a specific constituency or business interest, such as physicians. [Our] physicians had to face this issue of how do you decide to move a service from one hospital to the other when you are working at one of those hospitals. [CEO, conversion hospital]

The other issue of ethics in trusteeship concerned board composition. Two trustees mentioned this when asked what issues of ethics had arisen in their board. In one hospital that served a mostly minority community, medical staff members charged the board with racial discrimination, a charge that gained credence because of the absence of any minority members on the board. Although our respondent questioned the motives of those who brought these charges, it was the matter that was recalled when the respondent was asked if there had been ethical issues in the board. The other instance involved a board that was directed by the health department to recruit minorities to their board in a merger situation. The nominating committee chair, whom we interviewed, believed that being required to apply criteria other than picking the best people was itself an ethical issue, though he added that they had recruited "good people" for the slots in question.

Ethics in Trusteeship

Trustees mentioned a wide array of topics when asked if their board had dealt with any ethical issues in the previous year (see table 5.4). We have grouped

Table 5.4.   Responses by Hospital to the Question "What Are the Two Most Important Issues the Board Has Dealt with in the Last Year?" (n = 22)

Most Important Decision	Urban (n = 11)	Suburban (n = 5)	Conversion (n = 6)	Total
Merger/affiliation	8	4	5	17
Finance	6	5	3	14
Expansion of facility	6	3	1	10
Administration	4	1	4	9
Changes in health care industry	5	1	1	7
Access	4	1	1	6
Services	2	0	1	3
Board	0	1	1	2
Conversion to for-profit	0	0	1	1

Note: We collected this information from each chief executive officer and trustee that we interviewed; because of the consistency among respondents from particular institutions, we present the data with the institution as the unit of analysis.

these into three broad categories—patient-related, mission-related, and business-related. Each category includes several different issues. The fact that these topics were mentioned in response to a question about whether the board had dealt with ethical issues should be kept in mind. Respondents may have felt that they *should* be able to say "yes" to such a question and may have been reaching to find topics to mention. Notably, few of these topics were mentioned when we asked CEOs and trustees to describe the two most important issues that the board had dealt with in the previous year.

Patient-Related Issues

Perhaps because of the growth of bioethics, respondents mentioned thirty-nine patient-related issues when asked about ethical issues dealt with by their boards. These included care of terminally ill patients (eight mentions, six hospitals); issues involving abortion and reproductive health services (six/four); patients' rights, such as privacy (mentioned twice from the same institution); the activities of the hospital ethics committee (eight/six); and other patient care incidents and issues (seventeen/ten), involving, for example, serious accidents, possible malpractice, or even sexual assaults. For the most part, the issues in question were matters about which the boards had received reports and were apparently not matters in which they had engaged in depth. As one CEO put it, "patient care issues come up from time to time," often in the context of reports from the CEO or hospital committees that were given to the board "for informational purposes and comments."

This does not necessarily mean that boards are complacent about these topics. Many trustees said that they wanted their hospital to have good policies and procedures for dealing with difficult patient care decisions. Their comments generally suggested that they believed that their institution indeed had such procedures, which they often described when the topic of ethics was mentioned. For example, when asked whether there were ethical issues with which the board had dealt in the past year, the board chair of an urban hospital said: "[We deal with] what every hospital is dealing with: quality-of-life and life support issues [regarding] the terminally ill. Board members are members of the ethics committee and through their participation, they've all seen the extent to which they actually need such a committee." A board member from another institution told us of the only ethical issue that he recalled: "[Our board] hasn't seen much in the way of ethical breaches, [but] there was a plastic surgeon that was engaged in some improper activities. He was dealt with in a forthright manner [by the appropriate committee]." In sum, in many institutions board members—because of service on the specialized committees that dealt with bioethical and medical staff issues or because of briefings given to board members—were aware of bioethical issues arising in the hospital, as with the following board chair in a community hospital:

> Most [ethical issues] are dealt with by the committee and then are reported to and confirmed by the board. One issue was the development of a policy on how to deal with a Seventh-Day Adventist that refused to have blood transfusions. Another issue was the decision to change the rule that says that if a person should collapse outside the hospital, they have to be brought in by ambulance. Instead, they would just walk out and get them. Every department has a working ethics committee that reports to the board ethics committee, which then passes those reports on to the full board.

At some institutions, board members showed no awareness of ethical issues or the hospital committees. In several instances, the CEO would describe these matters when we asked about ethical issues, while board members at the same institution indicated that the board had dealt with no ethical issues. Clearly, institutions differ regarding whether they treat bioethical issues that arise within the hospital's walls as subject matter about which board members should be aware. And beyond having board representation on ethics committees and including significant issues as part of the routine reports to the board, few institutions appeared to treat bioethics and patient care issues as matters of importance for the board. However, there were exceptions to this generalization, as the following examples show:

> [We have] talked about palliative care and how you deal with pain. This has been discussed at the committee level, at the board level, and at trustee retreats. Doc-

tors are basically taught to keep people alive. We had a presentation to the board about the right to die with dignity and without pain. The board received this information and supported it. And now, we are going to be teaching our students and doctors with these goals in mind. [Chair, major teaching hospital]

We had an active discussion at our last board meeting. There was a patient who died in the ER [emergency room] whose death may have been due to an accidental administration of medication. The debate centered on whether the family should be told. The decision was no. The question came up because an empty vial of the medication was found on the patient's bed after she was moved. There was no other evidence that she had received the medication, and the timing of the death indicated that she had not. The hospital reported the death to the medical examiner's office, saying it might have been an accidental death. The medical examiner's office chose not to pursue it further. The decision not to tell the family was based on the fact that the medical evidence pointed away from administration of the drug. [Trustee, teaching hospital]

The institutions in which patient-related issues were described in the most detail were Catholic hospitals, particularly those that had been engaged in decisions regarding mergers with other institutions. Church teachings on issues pertaining to abortion and end-of-life decision making were emphasized, as were mission-related considerations regarding care of the poor. Many trustees in both Catholic and Jewish hospitals referred to religious teachings and traditions as providing an important ethical or moral compass that influenced the ways that trustees thought about how their institution should be run.

Mission-Related Issues

In response to our question regarding "ethical issues that their board had considered," our respondents mentioned twenty-three issues that pertained to the mission of their institution, particularly regarding community needs and the problem of indigent care. The topics mentioned included a decision whether to stay in the city or to relocate the hospital:

- decisions regarding availability of specialized services to meet community needs;
- a decision whether to help a nearby struggling institution;
- whether to permit two standards of care—for rich and poor people— within the hospital;
- making sure that the hospital is not turning away patients who need help;
- tensions between commitment to the hospital versus commitment to the community in trying to assure the financial soundness of the institution;
- trying to represent fairly the hospital's different constituencies (medical staff, employees, populations of different communities served by the hospital), regardless of one's bias or connections;

- deciding to close facilities that were losing money or in need of major capital infusions;
- deciding whether to sell to a for-profit firm; and
- resource allocation decisions, either in ordinary situations or regarding the use of the proceeds of the sale of the hospital.

Eight respondents mentioned mission-related issues that arose in situations involving mergers and sales of the hospital.[8] These are among the most difficult issues about which we heard:

> It looks like we will be doing a full asset merger with [two other hospitals]. Mission compatibility is our primary concern; we exist to serve a very needy population. [CEO, urban community hospital]

> Ethics are implicitly discussed in terms of our commitment to the community and how to maintain it. Questions include who is going to own the hospital and how to protect community control of the institution. [CEO, urban community hospital]

> Ethical issues? I think of them primarily as survival issues. But maybe ethical is "what is our responsibility to the community?" That was certainly a factor in our decision to go ahead with the [deal to help another hospital]. [Chair, urban community hospital]

> The merger with a Catholic hospital presented a number of ethical issues. The agreement calls for us not to be governed by the ethical and religious directives of the Catholic Church. But there was a lot of discussion about how the community would respond to a relationship with a Catholic facility and whether there would be any indirect influence to do things that we would not normally do or restrict things that we would not normally restrict. And what it will mean for us in the long run and the short run. [CEO, nonurban community hospital]

Three respondents replied to our question about ethical issues by referring to the ethos of their institution: in terms of sensitivity to how patients and employees are treated, protecting the "culture and heritage" of the institution, and faithfulness to values.

The close relationship between mission-related issues and business-related issues can be seen in this trustee's description of a recent decision of the board:

> When we were considering whether or not to have a hospice, we knew from day one it was going to lose X hundred thousand dollars a year, because reimbursement was just insufficient and that if we were going to have a hospice, the board would have to undertake to raise an endowment fund of $400,000. And they debated it and decided it was something we just had to do. [Chair, urban teaching hospital]

Business and Medical Staff Decisions

A group of some twenty-nine responses to our question about ethical issues with which their board had dealt pertained to business decisions. Although these responses shade over into mission-related matters, they were not so framed by our respondents. Examples pertained to the dangers to the institution of taking on additional debt; how to handle patients in the admissions office who come to a rehabilitation facility without a proper referral from a physician; how to handle downsizing and layoffs; the extent of salary differences from top to bottom of the institution; deciding whether overpayments identified in the hospital's compliance program should be returned ("It made for an interesting discussion when you tell your board that you just wrote a check for $200,000 back to Medicare. On the one hand, they are very proud that they are an ethical organization; on the other hand, it is a bit of a surprise, the magnitude of these things."); and having a strong corporate compliance program to assure that the institution does not violate regulations and the law.

Another large group of responses (fourteen) pertained to the medical staff—a doctor with a drug problem, unspecified "unethical behavior" by a physician; situations with physicians who have lost their licenses; issues in disciplining and occasionally removing a doctor from the staff; doctors' "behavior in the performance of their duty"; dealing with a "very contentious doctor" who the CEO feared would physically attack him; dealing with a staff member who fraudulently sued a restaurant for serving contaminated food (when he was responsible for the contamination himself); fraud-and-abuse concerns in contracting arrangements between the hospital and certain physicians; credentialing and quality issues; and how physicians handle cases with poor outcomes. All of these were mentioned as ethical issues with which the board had dealt.

THE GLOBAL VIEW OF ETHICS

Five respondents answered our question regarding whether their board had dealt with ethical issues by observing that all issues that came before the board were, in some sense, ethical issues. Here are some examples of how they made this important point.

> Probably every issue we face has an ethical aspect. If we weren't cognizant of the fact that we represent the community and the delivery of health care needs that it expects and requires, then our ethical responsibility would require it. . . . If we make decisions improperly or without proper information, in effect we've hurt these people in terms of access, quality, and comfortability of receiving care, and then ethically we have not begun to do our responsibility as trustees of health. [Trustee, nonurban community hospital]

I think every issue we deal with is an ethical issue. If you're adopting a budget, that's an ethical issue. How much money do you allocate to the emergency room? How much money is available for unreimbursed care? How do you take care of the uninsured? When you decide you're going to let some people go, those are ethical decisions. I think it's hard to separate out ethics from any decision facing a board today in any hospital. We're literally dealing with the most fundamental ethical issues that we have. Care for the sick and needy—I don't know how you can get more fundamental than that. There are other critical issues that have to be addressed. Do you treat people differently because they can pay? Do you treat people differently because they're on Medicaid as opposed to private insurance? I can tell you from the very beginning; [this hospital] has always been committed to one level of care. It just doesn't matter. We spent $60 million to take all of our clinics out of the hospital setting and move them into a magnificent facility on [location]. And when you go to see your doctor you're sitting in the same waiting room and you see the same people and you have the same beautiful ambiance, whether you're insured, whether you're an illegal alien, whether you've got Aetna or Oxford or you're paying out of your own pocket. It doesn't matter. [Chair, urban medical center]

Every issue becomes an ethical issue in light of the fact that you are serving the public with health care. The board tends to view many decisions as having ethical implications, including how faithful we are to our values, and how do we spend our money. If we need to downsize, we need to do so ethically, not to protect certain interests. We need to make sure that every department shares in the burdens. [Trustee, urban community hospital]

TENSIONS BETWEEN SOCIAL AND ECONOMIC VALUES

Many trustees that we interviewed experienced a tension between social and economic values in decisions regarding the hospital. This tension was highlighted in their responses to our questions as to whether their board had made any decisions in the past year "that could not be justified in terms of the economic interests of their hospital."

Some trustees seemed to feel that they would be confessing irresponsibility if they answered affirmatively. As one trustee said, "We try not to, but it happens." In most institutions, some (but not all) respondents indicated that their board had *not* made any decisions in the previous year that could not be justified in terms of the institution's economic interests, while other trustees from the same institutions gave us examples of just such decisions.

Conversely, some respondents seemed to think that a positive answer was correct for this question. Thus, at least some respondents from a majority of the hospitals in our New York–area sample indicated that their board had made a decision that could not be justified in economic terms. However, when asked for an example, they either could not think of any or they described a decision that they explained could be justified in business terms. For example, one trustee cited the decision to marge with a money-losing hospital, but then said that while it might appear that this merger was against the hospital's economic interest, the real purpose was to strengthen the hospital's economic position and would thus have a long-term economic payoff.

Judging from the interviews in our New York–area sample, boards commonly make decisions that they believe cannot be justified in terms of the hospital's best economic interests. At least one respondent from virtually every hospital in our New York–area sample provided at least one example of a decision that their board had made in the previous year that could not be justified in terms of the hospital's economic interest. Most examples pertained to decisions to maintain the hospital's commitment to providing uncompensated care to uninsured patients, decisions to establish or maintain money-losing services that were either used by low-income people or that were necessary (though unprofitable) to maintaining the hospital's ability to stay on the cutting edge of excellence, or decisions to maintain the commitment to research and training.

Sources of Guidance on Ethical Issues

The growth in the field of bioethics and its associated case law has increased the availability of sources of guidance to physicians and others who are faced with ethically difficult clinical decisions. Might bioethics be able to guide boards regarding institutional policies and strategies?

Most decisions made by trustees have received little ethical analysis to date, and few sources of guidance are now available for trustees regarding the ethical content of their decision making. Although we did not explore this question systematically, the sources of guidance mentioned by the trustees that we interviewed were: the principles of financial analysis and decision making; hospital mission statements, which in some (but not most) institutions are looked to for ongoing guidance, or a trustee's general sense of the hospital's mission and traditions; and a trustee's internalized sense of values and ethics. There were only occasional references to ethical principles in our interviews. These mostly pertained to the standards that the institution should pursue in providing patient care (mostly beneficence-related principles), and not to principles such as fairness or justice that might inform the kinds of resource-allocation decisions with which trustees are engaged.

General Conclusions

Governance by voluntary boards is both a great strength and potential weakness of the nonprofit hospital. We encountered boards that were obviously enormously talented, and board members who were highly engaged. We also visited institutions that had gotten into great difficulty in part because of failures in governance for which no self-corrective mechanism seemed to exist.

CEOs and trustees do not ordinarily see boards' responsibilities and decisions as having an ethical component. Respondents were commonly puzzled and struggled for an answer when asked if their board had dealt with any ethical issues in recent years. For many respondents, the term "ethical issue" carried a connotation of something having gone awry, as if having ethical issues arise in the board context meant that something (e.g., a serious conflict of interest) was wrong. (It is worth noting that respondents at five of the twenty-two institutions mentioned that their board had had serious conflict-of-interest problems, generally in the past.) Nor do board members use the vocabulary of ethics or refer to ethical principles in trying to resolve the issues they face. It was also striking that the issues mentioned in response to our question about ethical issues included few of the same mentioned in response to our later question about the "most important issues" with which their board had dealth in the previous year or so. Although there were important exceptions, most trustees and CEOs whom we interviewed seem to view matters of ethics as something quite distinct from, or peripheral to, the core activities or responsibilities of their board of trustees.

Yet it was abundantly clear that the decisions hospital boards of trustees make frequently have ethical dimensions and that these dimensions are a significant part of boards' deliberations regarding a wide variety of issues.[9] The fact that factors other than strictly business considerations are part of trustees' work had almost a "taken for granted" quality among many of the trustees we interviewed, perhaps because they generally had a clear understanding of the history, values, and mission of their institution or of charitable organizations in general. It is of course impossible for us to judge from our interviews how the tacit understandings of these matters actually play out in board deliberations.

Our interviews also revealed some fundamental ambiguities of ethical significance in the role of the hospital trustee. One pertains to whether it is legitimate for trustees to view themselves as serving in a representational capacity or to advocate for a particular interest in the board's deliberations. This implies a political model of the board of trustees, which may be incompatible with the basic duties of loyalty and fidelity. Some of the trustees we interviewed saw themselves as protecting particular interests, sometimes stating this in terms of adding balance to a board that was otherwise overly concerned with other (usually financial) matters. A related complexity arises in the increasingly common practice of physicians (and, presumably, CEOs, though that issue did not arise in our interviews) on the board. More than most board members, they may be directly affected by board decisions. The question is whether the fact that the resulting conflict of interest is not disguised renders it ethically acceptable.

Another area of ethical ambiguity experienced by trustees came to light when we asked trustees whether their board had made decisions that could not be justified in terms of their organization's best interest. Most seemed reluctant to acknowledge that their board had made such decisions. This suggests, we believe, that trustees may experience ethical tension between their obligations to see that the hospital adheres to a charitable mission and their stewardship responsibilities regarding a set of assets.

Another area of ambiguity regarding the trustees' roles concerned whether the trustees' obligations pertain to the best interests of the institution or the best interests of the community served by the institution. Although this issue arose in decisions regarding the sale or conversion of an institution (as is described in our companion chapter 10 below), it may also arise in other circumstances—the lengths to which an institution will go to best a competitor, the extent to which an institution will work with competing institutions to meet community needs, and how resources are allocated toward services that meet important needs but do not provide an economic return. As a related issue trustees should see themselves as representatives of the community, doing what they believe the community wants, or as independent agents using their best judgment in the interests of the institution or community.

The field of bioethics has a well-established set of concepts and principles with which to confront difficult problems of what to do with regard to a wide variety of ethical problems. Boards of trustees are working with no such set of concepts and principles. As a result, there are no consistent approaches to analyzing difficult problems, to identifying what problems should be dealt with by boards and which ones by management, or to determining what information is needed to make certain kinds of decisions or carry out ongoing oversight responsibilities. Yet many of the people we interviewed were deeply reflective of the responsibilities with which they were entrusted. An ongoing challenge for those who are concerned with the future of our hospitals and the role of governance therein is how to generalize the exemplars who recognize that all decisions made by hospital boards are, at their heart, ethical decisions.

NOTES

1. Rosemary Stevens, *In Sickness and in Wealth: The American Hospital in the Twentieth Century* (New York: Basic Books, 1999).

2. Academic Medical Centers and Teaching hospitals were defined according to Association of American Medical Colleges criteria.

3. For conversion hospitals, we focused on the CEO and board members at the time the decision was being made regarding the reorganization or sale of the hospital.

4. Because the CEO and/or chair selected the trustees to be interviewed, we may have been steered away from board members with dissenting views about important matters. Furthermore, our selection criteria regarding interest in clinical care, finance, and community may have led us to board members with the greatest responsibilities, experience, skills, and dedication.

5. In a few instances, particularly when travel from New York was involved, the research team separated to do two interviews at the same time. In one instance, the board chairs of two hospitals that had merged insisted on being interviewed jointly.

6. It is worth noting that only one trustee suggested that trustees' responsibilities included helping the institution to grow.

7. This question was asked of only eighty-nine CEOs and trustees because it was added to the survey after our first interviews had been done.

8. The question regarding ethical issues was not asked at most of the institutions contemplating for-profit sales, because the respondents knew before we came that we were interested both in ethics and in discussing their deliberations regarding the sale.

9. As we have indicated, the most important issues involved business decisions with very deep implications for the institution involving mergers, affiliations, or sales of the institution. The issues involved in these decisions are addressed in chapter 10 of this volume.

PART II

Ethical Perspectives

6

THE TRUSTEES OF NONPROFIT HOSPITALS

Dealing with Money, Mission, and Medicine

William F. May

America has relied heavily upon voluntary communities and nonprofit institutions for its flourishing as a nation. As far back as the 1830s, Alexis de Tocqueville referred to the vigor of voluntary communities as the distinctive feature of American society. John Nason aptly referred to the boards and staff members of nonprofit institutions and voluntary communities as "public servants." That characterization may surprise those who prefer to consign these groups to the "private sector," reserving the term "public" exclusively for officials who serve the government. But board members and leaders of nonprofit institutions, along with business leaders and government officials, cumulatively wield immense public power that fatefully affect millions of people. After government and business, nonprofit institutions constitute what Nason and others have called the "third sector" in American life.

TEMPTATIONS AND QUANDARIES

In their role as public servants, trustees and leaders in the third sector face at least two basic kinds of moral problems: temptations and quandaries. In the case of temptations, a clear distinction exists between right and wrong; but the public servant is tempted to do the wrong thing. Obviously, politicians betray their public identity when they wield power and money for merely private purposes. Shakespeare's Henry V recognized and rejected this temptation when he took up the public duties of the crown and recognized that he must break with his old friend Falstaff, who would treat the crown as a convenient windfall enriching their private life together as cronies. Similarly, prohibitions in trustee ethics against self-dealing and cronyism follow ethically from the need to sustain the public integrity of the enterprise. The actions of board members must be disinterested rather than self-interested. Otherwise, board members compromise their core identity as trustees.

Legal prohibitions against "interested" actions that violate the fiduciary responsibilities of board members and officers fall technically under the duty of loyalty. The law has most fully specified and enforced the duty of loyalty in the for-profit sector. As Harvey J. Goldschmid has written: "Fraud, self-dealing, misappropriation of corporate opportunities, improper diversions of corporate assets, and similar matters involving conflicts between a director's or officer's interest and the corporation's welfare are considered under duty of loyalty statutes and caselaw."[1] Clearly, nonprofit institutions have a similar right to expect from their trustees and officers the fulfillment of the duty of loyalty.

A second set of temptations fall under what the law has defined as the duty of care, that is, prohibitions against neglect and mismanagement. When trustees neglect and officers mismanage their duties of care to an institution, they have violated duties where a clear distinction exists between right and wrong. But they may not have done so to serve their own interests. Neglect and management may be "disinterested" but still very wrong.

The American Law Institute has specified these duties in detail for boards of directors in the for-profit sector (e.g., selecting managers and evaluating their performance and reviewing financial objections and corporate plans). Such duties of care have not usually been so sharply etched for boards of trustees in the nonprofit sector (other than the necessity for fund-raising). Still, a distinction exists between right and wrong when persons accept membership on a nonprofit board and neglect their duties of care.

The staffs and board members of nonprofit institutions face a second and larger range of ethical issues, which I would characterize as quandaries. A quandary, as opposed to a temptation, does not confront us with a clear choice between right and wrong but rather with an unavoidable conflict between competing goods or evils. Whatever choice the conscientious trustee makes, he or she faces the curtailment of some good or the imposition of some evil.

Trustees face such vexing moral quandaries whenever they engage in setting or approving institutional priorities. Where will scarce health care dollars go? To take care of AIDS patients or to establish a prenatal counseling center for pregnant teenagers? And if some money goes to both programs, how much for each? All decisions about priorities in the midst of contending needs and limited resources pose ethical quandaries. In this sense, Sargent Shriver observed that almost all questions reaching his brother-in-law's desk as president of the United States asked for an ethical judgment from President John Kennedy. Just so, trustee decisions about priorities call for ethical judgment. However, board members can obscure for themselves the moral import of those decisions when they think of themselves as merely "doing the budget."

In attempting to resolve quandaries, we usually make appeals to general moral principles, such as beneficence (doing good), nonmalficence (doing no harm), respect for patient autonomy, and justice (fairness in the distribution of benefits and harms). But appeal to the general principle of doing good does not settle the particular case of which good or goods, among competing goods, shall be supported—care for AIDS patients, or prenatal counseling for teenagers. Furthermore, the four principles often conflict in the specific case. One person's boon may be another's bane and still another's bone of contention. The principles of doing good, respect for autonomy, doing no harm, and acting fairly can conflict. Unfortunately, no philosopher or theologian can supply in advance a hierarchical list of goods and principles that will relieve trustees of the necessity of deciding how they shall be weighted in the specific case. Duties do not conveniently arrange themselves in a permanently valid hierarchy to resolve all quandaries.

Thus, board members will need to bring to the table not simply general principles but also virtues that will help resolve disputes. The virtue of practical wisdom surely heads the list. No set of abstract criteria for making decisions will do more than set one along the path. A trustee needs a practical wisdom that will attend patiently to the specifics of a case rather than operate deductively and repetitively from a favorite idea. A trustee also needs sufficient courage to face vexing issues that might more conveniently be swept aside, and yet enough humility not to blow the bagpipes too loudly and self-righteously for his or her own cause. The resilience of an organization surely depends upon maintaining civility between advocates of competing proposals as a given controversy makes its way up through the organization to its board.

THE QUANDARY OF QUANDARIES

The chief ethical quandary behind all other quandaries confronting the trustees of a nonprofit health care institution today is the never-ending tension between its mission objectives and the fiscal stringencies of the bottom line. We confuse thought on this tension if we relegate ethics to one sphere and economics to the other. Health care is a fundamental good, but it is not the only fundamental good; it perforce competes with many other fundamental goods for scarce resources, and therefore cost-effective management is a moral responsibility and not just an economic necessity.

Not-for-profit as well as for-profit institutions must attend to the bottom line: the one for the sake of its mission, the other to ensure its profits. If the trustees of a nonprofit institution ignore its deficits, they subject it to institutional martyrdom. They bear witness to its mission today but at the price of its demise tomorrow. By the same token, trustees cannot be so engrossed in the complexities of fiscal self-care as to marginalize the institution's mission. To strike the balance between the two is itself a moral issue. We miss the point when we compartmentalize the spheres of mission and finance.

We needed to draw the foregoing distinction between temptations and quandaries for two reasons. First, trustees tend to limit the arena of ethics to what we have called temptations, those behaviors obviously mired in wrongdoing. Hence trustees report that they seldom spend their time on moral issues—the burden of their work is financial. That limited view of ethics fails to address sufficiently the moral implications of allocative and financial decisions.

Second, the failure to distinguish temptations from quandaries glosses over the different meanings that the word "compromise" ought to carry in the two arenas. In the case of a temptation, where the trustee faces a clear distinction between right and wrong and does the wrong thing, he or she "compromises" in the sense of violating his or her core identity as a trustee. In the case of a quandary, where the trustee, in a world of scarce resources and clamorous needs for services, strikes off the best possible compromise, he or she fulfills rather than defects from his or her core responsibility as a trustee. Unfortunately, in the heat of fierce competition between advocates for rival uses of funds, good-faith differences of judgment can lead to suspicions that a trustee has in bad faith neglected or mismanaged his or her responsibilities. The recognition that trustees and officers face not simply moral temptations but also quandaries helps at once to subject quandaries to moral criticism while extracting some of the poison from the atmosphere of such criticism.

The Derivation of Mission in Health Care

We have identified the tension between mission and money in health care, but we have not yet attended to the question of the mission's origin. Some assume that the institution receives its mission exclusively and externally from the sponsoring religious or philanthropic agencies that formed and help sustain it. This view of the origin of the mission overlooks the possibility that the mission also derives internally from the very nature of the professions of nursing and medicine. If the constraints of the mission derive solely from external agencies, then for-profit health care institutions are free, like any other for-profit firm, to maximize profits.

Indeed, as free marketers argue, a for-profit hospital's board and officers have a fiduciary duty to stockholders to maximize profits. Any other mission evaporates. By the same token, if the constraints of mission for nonprofits derive solely from their external sponsoring agency, then trustees of nonprofit institutions will find themselves isolated in their own institutions (in the midst of doctors and nurses who may not have bought into that mission). Trustees may also find themselves eventually outgunned in the marketplace by the for-profits that operate with no such constraints upon their pursuit of market share.

We need then to ask ourselves what it means to profess medicine and whether that profession generates a mission internal to the practice of medicine irrespective of the sponsoring agency. If a mission defines a medical profession that does not simply depend upon the eleemosynary commitments of the sponsoring agency, then that mission may, to the degree that practitioners profess it, serve to level the playing field for both for-profits and nonprofits as they struggle in the marketplace. Further, this mission internal to the practice of medicine may well fit and reinforce the mission that is externally derived from a sponsoring nonprofit agency.

MONEY AND MEDICINE

Reflection on money and medicine must concede that medicine (and all other helping professions) rests on a complicated, double relationship with the marketplace: They grow and expand together in the modern world, and yet they differ (or ought to differ) in their essence. The professional, at least in part, belongs to the world of money. We sometimes distinguish the amateur from the professional in that the amateur does it for love and the professional does it for money. It would be a species of angelism to deny this fact. Yet the professional, who has one foot in the marketplace, also, purportedly, professes something else—beyond the bottom line. I turn now to explore the morally complex ties between money and the health care professions, which the boards of nonprofit and for-profit institutions alike must face.

The increased power of the professions in the modern world coincides and intertwines with the emergence of the modern marketplace and with the still later emergence of the winner in the marketplace, the modern, large-scale corporation.

I see the connections as follows. Aristotle once referred to the good community, the polis, as a community of friends, people who share needs and goals.

Aristotle's ideal city was quite small, small enough to be a community of well-known, familiar names and to engage every one (well, not exactly everyone; not women or slaves) in civic responsibilities. The city remained relatively small until the eighteenth century. This cameo scale let people in the city associate chiefly within the framework of family, neighbors, and friends. From the eighteenth century onward, the West and particularly the United States increasingly shifted from a community of neighbors to a society of strangers. (In Dallas, where I live now, the house-attached garage completes the process of separating the self from the neighbor. I drive home along an alley, flick the garage door open to avoid getting out of the car, park inside, and then flick the garage door shut and enter the kitchen. If children are out in their front yards playing, if neighbors are out mowing the grass, I would not know it. We live in a society of strangers—sometimes friendly strangers, but still strangers.)

How do persons in the modern setting connect? Mostly, not through shared interests, but through cash, which temporarily connects people who otherwise may share few common interests. Professionals are part of that platoon of paid strangers who partly substitute for the families, neighbors, and friends who provided services in earlier societies.

Aging patients (with their children in distant cities) now look to the physician and nurse as the fixed stars in their lives. Women look to obstetrician-gynecologist specialists rather than to the experienced aunt or the competent neighbor for assistance in birth. At one time, disputes were resolved through the mediation of friends and neighbors acquainted over a lifetime with the parties to a conflict. They now end up in the courts. Precisely because the doctor-patient relationship today chiefly connects strangers linked by money and because it points toward a desperately hoped-for favorable outcome, the relationship is increasingly unstable and, thus today, sometimes erupts into enmity. The disappointed patient resorts angrily to the court, which in its own right and turn is controlled by strangers to both parties; strangers attempt to bring closure to the disputes between strangers, with money at issue at every point.

Although the professions and the marketplace (and money) grew together in the modern world, the professional cannot be tidily equated with the seller of services in the marketplace. The professional has a double identity. He or she has one foot in the marketplace, being paid for work. But at the same time, he or she has a commitment transcending the marketplace.

We express this transcendence least satisfactorily by pointing to the aristocratic origins of the professional in the West. "Having a profession" provided a social location in life for the second, third, and fourth sons of aristocrats, who, in a society committed to primogeniture, could not inherit the land (the family property went exclusively to the eldest son), and yet who, as children of the aristocracy, could not submit to the vulgarities of the marketplace by working for a living. Thus the professions—the law, civil service, the military, and medicine—provided the great families with an honorable social location, a parking lot, for their surplus gentlemen.

A vestigial remnant of this aristocratic reserve persists in the professional complaints that money vulgarizes. Thus professionals should not advertise, least of all their fees, lest they tarnish the moral elegance of the honorarium. The courts, beginning with the Virginia decision in the 1970s, banned professional guilds from prohibiting advertising on the grounds that such prohibitions led to monopolistic price fixing. The cost of professional services rose much faster than the rate of inflation. Thus the professions, while invoking an ethic superior to the marketplace, in effect behaved in a fashion morally inferior to the marketplace. Understandably, the courts wanted to put a stop to this hypocrisy. But rampant advertising does make one wince. Money vulgarizes. "Two root canals for the price of one until the end of the month." Radial keratotomy at $1,250 an eye, with $500 off for the two procedures if you make your decision before you leave our seminar room." "If you need a lawyer's help on your traffic ticket, just dial 9-GOTCHA, credit cards accepted."

Recoiling from money matters, professionals daintily hand over to their office staffs the task of collecting money from their patients and clients so as not to brush up too close to cash.

But the polite conventions of professional billing do not fool. Professional schools increasingly require courses in business management; they enroll more students in purely elective courses than in professional ethics. Moreover, the social profile of the recruits for the professions has changed massively and for good social reasons. The professions no longer serve as the parking place for the younger sons of aristocrats but as the social escalator that carries the children of the working class upward—advancing those previously without clear public identities and often without resources, who need to earn their entire living from their profession. Thus the modern professional seems to have both feet planted in the marketplace.

The question grows more acute. Does the professional have any further identity that transcends the cash nexus? Is the professional simply a combination of technician plus entrepreneur, someone who sells a skill in the law, medicine, accounting, engineering, teaching, or pastoring? Or is the professional something more?

Roscoe Pound, the great jurist, sought to illuminate this further reach of professional identity by invoking the old religious term, a "calling." In an oft-quoted line, he said, "The term [profession] refers to a group . . . pursuing a learned art as a common calling in the spirit of public service—no less a public service because it may incidentally be a means of livelihood. Pursuit of the learned art in the spirit of public service is the primary purpose."[2]

Pound thus defines a profession as a calling, and he links a calling with the pursuit of the common good. The religious tradition of the West made this connection in its Scriptures as did William Perkins, a seventeenth-century Puritan who was influential on the American scene. He defined a calling as that "kind of life, ordained and imposed on man by God, for the common good."[3] So conceived, all lines of work, but especially those that serve goods basic to our common life, such as law, medicine, and religion, are callings and ought to contribute to the common good.

However, in our time the notion of a calling has tended to deteriorate into a career. A career refers to that wherein I invest myself, on the basis of scores on standardized achievement and placement tests—PSATS, SATS, GRES, LSATS, and MCATS—to pursue my own private goals. Etymologically, a career derives from the same root as a car. A career is an automobile, a self-driven vehicle through life, in and through which we enter into the public thoroughfares for the purposes of reaching our own private destinations.

But if a profession is a calling to serve a public good and not simply a vehicle for serving our own private, careerist aims for money and fame, then we have arrived at a second danger and temptation of money, more serious than the first.

Money not only vulgarizes; it also distracts. The moralist Alasdair MacIntyre distinguishes between the goods internal to a practice—such as the arts of lawyering, healing, and preaching—and the goods external to a practice—such as the fame or fortune that those practices may generate.[4] If someone chooses medicine or law, only for the prestige or the cash, he or she has lost the single-mindedness, the purity of heart, that allows all else to burn away as the practice shines through. The love of money and fame distracts; it focuses attention elsewhere. The professional loses that purity of heart, which the Epistle of James and later Søren Kierkegaard reminded the world, is "to will one thing."

In Kingsley Amis's 1954 novel Lucky Jim, an eccentric college history professor answers his telephone saying, "History here." What a wonderful line! Better than "Historian here" or "Dr. Toynbee here." "History here" points to the activity, pure and simple, not to the office or to the attainment of the person. Is that not what a distressed patient wants when calling the doctor about a baffling symptom? "Healing here." Is that not what the distressed client or parishioner needs when calling a lawyer or priest? "Sanctuary here."

But money distracts the professional and the institution in which he or she works from what should be his or her single-minded professional purpose (the client's welfare) by focusing a wall-eye on some external good.

Money corrupts. Eventually, a distracted focus on the goods external to a practice corrupts the practice itself. The actor interested only in Nielsen television ratings and the advertising revenue they generate repeats the tricks of the trade that worked last week, and at length the show deteriorates into a series of running gags, clichés that corrupt the internal good of the original performance.

The specific corruption of money in the case of the professional transaction can be stated as follows. A marketplace transaction, as distinct from a professional exchange, presupposes two self-interested and relatively knowledgeable parties engaged in the act of buying and selling. Each party attempts primarily to protect his or her own self-interest. The seller does not feel particularly constrained to watch out for the buyer's interests and well-being. That is up to the buyer who, by comparative shopping and other means, has ways of becoming knowledgeable.

But a basic asymmetry exists in the relation of the professional to his or her client. The professional possesses knowledge (and the power that knowledge generates), while the troubled client is often too ignorant, powerless, anxious, and dependent to protect his or her interests. A medical crisis, moreover, usually leaves little time for comparative shopping, even if the patient knew how to assess the professional's skills. Patients, students, clients, and parishioners cannot readily obey the marketplace warning, caveat emptor—buyer beware. Their lack of knowledge and their neediness require that the professional exchange take place in a fiduciary setting of trust that transcends the marketplace assumptions about two wary bargainers. The importance of this trust should determine our view of what the professional has to sell.

I am very fond of a Volvo automobile and thus have often walked into a Volvo showroom, but I have never yet had a salesperson say to me, "Professor May, do you really need this car? In the total economy of your life, as a professor, wouldn't it make more sense for you to trot across the highway and buy a Toyota Tercel at half the price?" Instead, the salesperson does his best to serve his own self-interest and sell me the car. When I enter the showroom, I am a pork chop for the eating. That is part of the game.

But if I visit a physician, I must be able to trust that he or she sells two items, not one. First the physician, to be sure, sells a procedure. But second, the doctor must also offer a professional judgment that I need the treatment offered. The surgeon is not simply in the business of selling hernia jobs. He or she also sells a cold, detached, disinterested, unclouded judgment that I need that wretched little procedure. If the surgeon sells me more operation than I need, the surgeon abuses his or her disproportionate power and poisons the professional relationship with distrust. Instead of sheltering, the surgeon takes advantage of the distressed, reducing me merely to a profit opportunity. And if I discover the surgeon pushing his or her own interests at my expense, I will resent him or her for exploiting my ignorance and powerlessness. Herein lies the ground for all professional strictures against conflicts of interest.

Until recently, under the prevailing fee-for-service system in medicine, money has worked, on the whole, to create temptations to overtreat patients. Coupled with third-party insurance coverage, the system has led to the overuse of medical services and sometimes to the abuse of patients, pummeled as they were by often irrelevant or unnecessary tests.

However, money can corrupt the medical exchange by creating incentives not only for excessive treatment under a fee-for-service system but also for inadequate treatment under prepayment systems. Physicians profit under many prepayment systems from the surplus of income over medical costs.[5] This time, money tempts physicians to do too little rather than too much. One moves from the sins of the overbearing to the sins of the underbearing. Under either payment system, runaway self-interest—avarice—can find a way to corrupt.

In the current environment, differences surely exist between for-profit and nonprofit institutions; but both types of institutions face the temptation to weaken the professional's identity with the well-being of the patient. Both must contend, as we noted above, with the pressures of the marketplace—one, to make a profit; the other, simply to survive. The nonprofit institution, encumbered with a mission to serve poor people or to support research, can find itself faced with the prospect of institutional decline, demolition, or conversion. In both institutional settings, obsession with the bottom line can take the oxygen out of the air of professionals and what they profess.

Money distorts, as well as corrupts, distracts, and vulgarizes the professional relationship. That claim requires us to identify a further way, in addition to its disinterestedness, in which the professional exchange should differ from a marketplace transaction.

The commercial transaction between buyer and seller seeks to gratify the buyer's wants. The professional exchange should be, when circumstances require, transformational, and not merely transactional.[6] The practitioner in the helping professions must respond not simply to the client's self-perceived wants but also to his or her deeper needs.

The patient suffering from insomnia often wants simply the quick fix of a pill. But if the physician goes after the root of the problem, he or she may have to help the patient transform the habits that led in the first place to the symptom of sleeplessness. The physician is slothful if he or she dutifully jumps to acute care but neglects preventive medicine.

Most of the incentives in conventional fee-for-service medicine favor acute care, at the expense of preventive, rehabilitative, long-term, and terminal care; they favor physical, at the expense of mental, health care. The physician who hands patients what they want—sleeping pills—gets them out of the office faster. The physician's basic office costs of receptionist, secretary, and nurse come out roughly the same, whether he or she handles more or fewer patients. Thus the temptations are great to become an artful people mover.

To question a patient about his or her deeper problem takes time. "What gives with your Atlas syndrome that you can't let go of the world for seven hours? Have you thought about your perfectionist tendencies that make you lie in bed at night, reliving painfully the gaffes of the previous day or worrying about the overload of duties that fill the morrow?" Such counseling takes time. It demands effective teaching of the patient, and teaching is slow boring through hard wood.

Finally, money excludes. It sets up barriers. Money opens doors, but usually only to those who can pay for a key. Those who cannot pay their way into the marketplace cannot acquire the good. That arrangement works out acceptably enough in the purchase of optional commodities—like a portable earphone radio, a tie, or a scarf—but professionals presumably generate and offer not optional commodities but basic goods—goods needed for human security and flourishing. Without the good of medicine, people suffer a triple deprivation: the misery of their trouble, the desperation of no treatment, and the cruel proof on the part of the society that they do not really belong. The untreated ill, the undefended client, become aliens in their own land. Thus even while money leaps over and seeps under boundaries and enclaves, it also excludes and expels. The principle of universal access derives from the conviction that health care is a fundamental good, not an optional commodity. Universal access goes to the soul of health care reform.

In the foregoing, I have emphasized the loss imposed upon patients and society when the professional exchange diminishes altogether to a commercial transaction. What of the loss to professionals themselves? What good internal to the practice of health care do professionals forfeit to the degree that they yield to the enticements and hazards of the marketplace and especially those proffered by the winner in the modern marketplace, the large organization?

The good internal to the practice of doctoring is the art of healing. Medicine and nursing surely draw on science in the diagnosis and treatment of disease. However, we cannot adequately describe medicine as an applied science. When we interpret and organize the profession simply as an applied science, we lose the soul of the activity. A scientist traffics in universals. A scientific hypothesis prescinds from the complexity of the universe; it selects for description a particular set of recurrent phenomena, isolated from all the variables in which they might be embedded, and seeks a generalization that covers the phenomena under scrutiny and that provides the basis for targeted interventions.

Whereas the scientist thus traffics in universals, the artist instead offers a concrete universe—Lear's universe, Antigone's world, the world of Michelangelo's Pieta. About the abstraction of the scientist's formula, H_2O, the poet William Butler Yeats once complained, "I like a little seaweed in my definition of water." We must define healing as an art because the individual patient whom it serves does not simply illustrate a general scientific principle into which that patient entirely disappears. The patient lives in his or her own full-bodied person with a particular history and universe. For instance, one patient's diabetes may more or less illustrate a generalization about the particular disease. But we cannot tidily abstract the host from the disease or the disease from the host. To diagnose the disease, we must discern the person; treating the disease and helping the patient face his or her disease require knowing his or her habits, world, pressures, and strains. These complex undertakings surely draw on science, but the physician must artfully marshal the resources to heal rather than merely treat; to help discern, mend, and make whole the universe embodied in the person of each patient, rather than prescind from that universe to handle a detail that fits and confirms an abstract rule.

Institutional pressures today favor interpreting medicine as a retailable, applied science. The reduction of medicine to an applied science fits conveniently into the current corporatization of health care. If doctoring merely applies science or technical expertise then one can diagnose, treat, and heal at a distance—the very considerable distance of a toll-free telephone number, for instance, with a case manager at the other end of the phone with a recipe book in hand. The doctor becomes retailer and dispenser of interventions authorized elsewhere.

But, as a psychiatrist remarked to me: Every thoughtful psychiatrist knows that the better you get to know a patient, the more difficult it is to classify him under one of the diseases listed in the *Diagnostic and Statistical Manual of Mental Disorders*. The patient does not conveniently vanish into the scientist's universal. The doctor uses science, but healing also requires practical wisdom in bringing science artfully to bear in restoring harmony to the patient's universe. That healing is the end purpose of doctoring.

Such doctoring takes time; whereas managed care requires the new coercive art of saving time. The technique of moving people rapidly through a system is a modern art form of which Walt Disney was master. The Disney theme parks enclose an expensive piece of finite space and face chronic core costs. The parks make their money by moving people through them efficiently, rapidly, and happily. (I belong to a golf club that learned its lesson from Disney. The corporation that owns and runs the club has kept trees to a minimum. Why? Trees block golf shots; and in the fall, they also shed leaves and make balls hard to find; thus trees slow up the game. More trees mean that golf scores will be higher, players less happy, the playing time longer, and the course unable to support as many members and thus yield as large a profit to the owners.)

After I offered some of these remarks in the course of grand rounds at a distinguished teaching hospital, my hosts reported that the hospital had invited in as consultants just a few weeks earlier two experts from the Disney Corporation to learn how to hustle people happily through the system. Today we talk somewhat inelegantly of the commodification and the corporatization of health care; increasingly, this commercialization and corporatization ends in its Disneyfication.

So much for the subject of money as it vulgarizes, distracts, corrupts, distorts, excludes, and thus endangers the integrity of the professions. I have not offered these warning signals about money to dismiss it but rather to let money do its proper yet limited work—as it feeds and motivates professionals, as it connects them to the stranger, and as it mobilizes their resources and talents in the huge institutions where they most often work. Money is a useful but unruly servant. We need to take care that it sustains rather than obscures what we profess on behalf of patients when we dare to cut, burn, or laser their bodies or advise them. What we profess ought to come down to what our patients surely hope for: "Healing here."

CONCLUDING REMARKS

In fulfilling their intramural role, hospital trustees, like doctors and nurses, must serve an institution that functions and survives, as best it can, in a double world. Trustees must be wall-eyed, as it were, keeping one eye on the bottom line, which they cannot ignore if the institution would survive, but attending with the other eye to the mission that derives in part from the intentions of donors and in part from the very nature of the good that the institution offers. Health care calls for a disinterested rather than self-interested response to the needs of patients; and it would elicit from practitioners and the institutions they serve the highest quality of patient care. Intramurally, the board has the task of cultivating the ethos required to make good on these purposes. The coherence of that ethos cannot be taken for granted. It often includes jostling, sometimes colliding, cultures of managers and administrators and doctors and nurses.

From the doctor's perspective, managers and trustees seem increasingly engaged in distorting the fundamental good that the institution offers. For the sake of the bottom line, they trim and shave on the range of services; they hem in patients with limits on treatment; and they have a hand on the elbows of doctors and nurses to hurry patients along through the system. In short, doctors increasingly complain that the institution and its managers are talking the oxygen out of the air that professors of medicine and nursing must breathe.

Meanwhile, the managers of institutions—both for-profit and nonprofit—have grounds for dismay. Doctors complain about market-driven institutions, while they themselves make many of their own decisions largely on the basis of recruitment bonuses, financial packages, office supports, perks, and fringe benefits. There is something unseemly about overestimating one's own ethical behavior while underestimating the ethics of others. Trustees attending to the moral culture of an institution, its mission or calling as it were, must help each constituency within it—professional and managerial—answer to the "better angels" of its nature. Fortunately, in this effort, the trustees of a nonprofit institution, if they carefully appoint and cultivate staff, should be able to appeal not only to the mission derived from external sponsoring bodies but also to the mission internal to the professions of medicine and nursing, and latent within the profession of those administrators called to manage the production and distribution of this fundamental human good.

A board of trustees also has an extramural role to play, which the very nature of health care as a fundamental human good lays upon the board. The importance of health care to human well-being cries out for a fulfillment beyond the intramural capacity of any institution to attain. The health care system as a whole needs to offer universal access and a comprehensive range of services. It needs to ensure the continuance of high quality through the support of medical education and the improvement of that quality through the support of medical research. Through its allocations, a board of trustees can testify to the importance of these larger goals, but only in a limited way do they lie within the reach of the institution's intramural resources. However, the board can serve as a powerful instrument through which the hospital can build alliances with other institutions to address health care needs beyond the reach of any one institution to solve.

While spending a sabbatical year as an observer at a tertiary care hospital, I visited one of its satellite neighborhood clinics and accompanied a modestly trained physician's assistant who made home visits to provide preventive and follow-up care for some of the clinic's patients. Before I set out on the rounds, the nurse who headed the clinic predicted that I would soon discover that poor housing ranked as the major health problem in the neighborhood. She was right. The hospital needed to reach out to other kinds of agencies to deal with the causes of health problems in that neighborhood. It had to build alliances with other institutions to address the health problems that grow apace beyond its walls. David H. Smith and others have warned of "mission creep," the danger that an institution will weaken if it loses its boundaries, the precision of clear-cut tasks. Still, the nonprofit institution can often make a difference in a threatened neighborhood if it plays out its role as an institutional citizen through the good offices of its board.

Nonprofits will also have to band together and think through dispassionately the question of the government's regulatory and financial roles if they hope to see society at large address at more than token levels the problems of universal and comprehensive health care. In the 1980s, for-profits did 50 percent of the health care business but only 6 percent of the charity work in Florida (a figure itself perhaps inflated by the practice of writing off deadbeats, who wriggled through the filter, as charity cases). A Catholic health care system in Florida found itself at a hopeless disadvantage trying to compete with the for-profits to stay afloat, while bearing, along with municipal hospitals, the full burden of giving universal access to health care. They could not compete in the long term if the for-profits accepted little responsibility for the nature of the fundamental good that they sell. The for-profits pay taxes, to be sure, but their taxes only very remotely and their profits only negligibly help meet the needs for universal access to health care or provide support for medical education and research. The nonprofits must do what they can symbolically to make good on the mission of medicine, but the ideals that their good works symbolize will not permit trustees to confine the duties of trusteeship wholly within the walls of the institution.

NOTES

1. Harvey J. Goldschmid, "The Fiduciary Duties of Nonprofit Directors and Officers: Paradoxes, Problems, and Proposed Reforms," *Journal of Corporation Law* 23, no. 4 (summer 1998): 646.

2. Roscoe Pound, *The Lawyers from Antiquity to Modern Times* (Saint Paul: West Publishing Company, 1953), 5.

3. William Perkins, "A Treatise of the Vocations or Callings of Men, with Sorts and Kinds of Them and the Right Use Thereof," in *Puritan Political Ideas*, ed. Edmund S. Morgan, (Indianapolis: Bobbs-Merrill, 1965), 35–59.

4. Alasdair MacIntyre, *After Virtue* (Notre Dame, Ind.: University of Notre Dame Press, 1981), 178.

5. Marc Rodwin, *Medicine, Money, and Morals* (New York: Oxford University Press, 1993), 56–94.

6. For an extended discussion, see William F. May, *Beleaguered Rulers: The Public Obligations of the Professional* (Louisville: Westminster John Knox Press, 2001), 27–85. The distinction between transactional and transformational relationships is discussed in James MacGregor Burns, *Leadership* (New York: Harper & Row, 1978).

TRUSTEES AND THE MORAL IDENTITY OF THE HOSPITAL

David H. Smith

I will argue that trustees should be the guardians of a hospital's moral integrity—meaning by that its fidelity to its mission, its standards for dealing with the professionals it works with and the patients it serves. Of course, those parties have moral responsibilities of their own, but I insist that the board has particular and irrevocable responsibilities for the institution itself.

I presuppose a broad definition of morality in which the main focus is on responsible behavior as determinative of the moral. I shall not be particularly concerned about standards for individual probity: honest dealing, avoiding conflict of interest, responsible fiscal management and the like. My omission of these topics does not mean that I regard those standards as unimportant. Quite the contrary. But focus on those issues too easily leads a board to think of its responsibilities in terms of "thou shalt nots"—of things that must be avoided. Though I agree that they must be avoided, I think that morality has a more positive and demanding component, as I shall try to explain.

This chapter has three sections. I begin by sketching the groundwork for the vision of trusteeship that drives what I have to say.[1] After that, I focus attention on some key features of hospitals as entrusted institutions. I conclude with reflections on the specific responsibilities of hospital trustees at the beginning of the twenty-first century.

What Is a Trustee, Morally Speaking?

Trusteeship is a form of relationship that arose in classical antiquity and the Middle Ages as a way of perpetuating ideals, ideas, visions, and property. The biblical term for this kind of relationship is usually translated "stewardship." The key idea is that the trustee takes responsibility for someone or something on behalf of someone else. In trusteeship, we can identify and distinguish what I am responsible for from the party to whom I am responsible. An example is that someone assumes responsibility for the investment and protection of money or property for someone else. What I am responsible for is the money, but I am responsible to those whom the money is supposed to benefit: my grandchild, friend, or mother.

In the simplest case, a trustee is chosen because the person who sets up the relationship believes that he or she will sustain the things in trust in ways that will maximally assist the beneficiary. Both what and for whom may be understood much more broadly, however. For example, in religious environmental ethics, it is often said that human beings have a responsibility to God for the natural environment, a responsibility that is also understood as a form of stewardship.

Before proceeding, we should notice that this triangulated notion of moral responsibility is different from that at work in many moral discussions of other issues. We often think of morality in two-party terms, focusing on the reciprocal rights and duties of parents and children, women and men, patients and physicians. Perhaps more of those relationships are best understood on the stewardship model than we usually suppose, but I don't want to take time to argue that thesis here. Instead, I mean to observe that tripartite responsibility or trusteeship is more complicated than two-party morality because of the separation between parties. For example, if I have a duty to my students to come to class, it is plausible to argue that they may release me from that duty. But if my duty to come to class and teach them is rooted in a commitment to someone or something else—my department, or college, or university, or God—then it is less clear that the students can let me off the hook. I am responsible for their education but I am not, in the last analysis, responsible to them.

Whatever the deficiencies of this way of looking at things as a pedagogical theory, it accurately captures some ideas that are at the heart of trusteeship. The trustee is responsible for providing certain goods and services for the welfare of the beneficiary, but he or she is responsible to the beneficiary only indirectly—that is, through the will or directive of the entruster. Responsibility to the beneficiary is mediated.

From this standpoint, it becomes apparent that trusteeship inevitably has an orientation to the past as well as to the future, because the trustee finds in the past the pivot on which his responsibilities turn. The glance at the past does not mean that trustees can never make major changes, but it does mean that maintaining coherence with the specifics of the entruster's history and identity is part of the job.

For example, if a hospital was founded by a religious community, that is a dimension of its identity to be taken seriously. We should not be worried because Jewish, Catholic, Methodist, or Adventist forebears might be startled at the things now done in hospitals bearing their names, as long as we can give an account of the sense in which those specific community identities remain valid. If such an account cannot be given, then the specific names should be dropped.

I have found it helpful to think of this aspect of trustee responsibility as a fidelity principle, referring to fidelity to the founding vision. The requirements of fidelity to that vision may change with the passage of time. (If circumstances did not change, there would be no need for the trustees.) But trustees are constrained by more than fidelity and change; their moral responsibilities are determined by principles of social justice.

Trustees must complement the fidelity principle with a commitment to the common good of the larger community of which their hospital is a part. The phrase "common good" is notoriously ambiguous, and I do not mean to use it to smuggle in a full-blown theory of justice. But the general point is very important.

Governance by nonprofit-sector trustees is an essential part of a free society because it enables a plurality of centers of power. We can imagine a different kind of society with all power to do good lodged in a central political apparatus. Such a society might be administratively efficient, but it would be potentially totalitarian, as it would have the power to enforce a narrow conception of the good life on the society's citizens. Against this, nonprofit trusteeship entails a greater degree of pluralism and support for competing visions of a good life.

There are limits, however, on the range of options that entrusted institutions may support by their actions, and I want to use the terms common good or social justice to name those limits. The vision of the good that a hospital board stands for must cohere with the perceived needs and sense of justice in a community, if the hospital is to be treated as a respected nonprofit organization within the community. Whatever its distinctive origins, a hospital is not at liberty to declare itself above the moral fray of argument about what is needed or just in a particular community at a particular time. Resources and good motives are not enough; what is done must really benefit the world into which the trustees have entered.

I do not mean to impose any particular agenda on the trustees at this point, only to argue that fidelity to a founding vision is insufficient for their guidance. In addition, they must look outward and to the future. They must make judgments about the health care needs of their community, and they must be prepared to revise their vision of the mission of the hospital with these new data in mind. Indeed, the crucial role of the board lies in this process of revision and reconciliation of historic mission and current need. A competent board must be a group able to take on this task, a task I can only describe as philosophical.

SPECIFYING NEEDS AND BUILDING ALLIANCES

Hospitals are differentiated from many other organizations because they have a commitment to health or, if one prefers, to providing health care. In this commitment, they contrast with colleges and universities, libraries, and symphony orchestras, which are primarily concerned with education, provision of information, and music. Of course any one hospital may well approach the pursuit of health from a distinctive perspective—Jewish, Catholic, or Methodist. But it calls itself a hospital because it claims to offer services that relate to health care needs.

The hospital board's role as custodian of changing mission is particularly important because health needs change. Change may occur when a new pathology develops, or it may happen because advances in medical research and technology enable treatment for a problem that has heretofore resisted attempts at cure or palliation. Our responsibilities to care for each other relate to what we can do to help. As therapies ranging from major surgeries to orthodontia and psychiatric care are developed, it may make sense to speak of someone as needing those procedures or medicines.

Hospital board life would be much simpler if boards could avoid the question of what forms of health care people most need. In contemporary American usage, the concept of need is, as Norman Daniels puts it, an "opportunistic" concept,[2] meaning that we tend to include a great range of preferences and desires under the rubric of need. A customer in a restaurant will say that he needs a martini; someone else may say he needs a Jaguar automobile. Need easily blurs into desire. We also have an unfortunate tendency to think of our own preferences as needs and those of others as wants or desires, or at any rate as optional.

The fact that needs change over time and that people disagree about what is needed does not mean that we cannot make judgments about needs. In fact, as writers with diverse agendas have claimed,[3] health needs relate to the capacity of human beings to function as human beings. Normal human functions include eating and breathing, eliminating waste, the ability to move, and the capacity to see, hear, and smell the world around us. They also include possession of psychic strength or balance sufficient to sustain a capacity to interact with others and one's environment.

These may not be the most apposite possible descriptors of the range of human biological and social functioning that should be included under the concept of health and health needs, but it is close enough for my purposes here. Beyond the crucial capacity to function as social animals, we have to say that health is a matter of degree. It makes sense to speak of a healthy person who has an artificial limb, suffers from a mental illness, or is confined to a wheelchair, but those persons are less healthy than others not so affected. Our goal should be to make persons as healthy as they can be.

I concede immediately that this is a very broad and vague statement about what health care needs are. Specifying priorities among various contenders for the most pressing health care needs is not easy, even in the simplest and most homogeneous communities. But the very fact that the concept of health care needs is indeterminate argues for identifying a group of people who will specify which of a long list of needs a particular hospital will try to meet in a particular time and place. If health care needs were always and everywhere the same, the need for trustee governance would be greatly reduced.

Beyond the fact that hospitals are dedicated to advancing a good that hospital trustees must specify, there is another important characteristic of hospitals that must be taken into account when we think of trustee responsibility. Hospitals exist in a symbiotic relationship with highly trained professionals, and they now relate to two of those groups in remarkably different ways. The first group is nurses. Although nurses are not shapers of hospital policy, they are characteristically the largest key group of hospital employees. But nurses are strongly pulled in other directions. Part of the pathos of nursing in early-twenty-first-century America is the number of masters to whom nurses are accountable: patients, hospitals, and physicians all claim very high levels of allegiance.[4] Conversely, nurses are increasingly well trained and militant, and hospitals must sustain high morale among them.

Physicians are at least as important, but the relationship is another story. Although the number of physicians employed by hospitals is rising, for the most part physicians remain independent professionals—albeit increasingly in group rather than solo practice.

Even when physicians are hospital employees, they retain great power because they are gatekeepers for the entire institution. Imagine a college or university in which individual faculty members did ad hoc admissions! It would never work. We have made some rough equivalent work—at least to a point— in the delivery of health care, but not without stress. In one community with which I am familiar, conflicts between powerful medical groups and the hospital administration are endemic. First one urologist wanted the hospital to purchase a lithotriptor, or to join in its purchase, and then to locate it in his suite of offices several miles from the hospital campus. A few years later, the largest and most distinguished group of internists in town decided to set up a large new suite of offices that would include several small operating theaters suitable for all but the most advanced cardiac procedures. They were aghast when the hospital offered exclusive privileges to two young invasive cardiologists who had separated from them.

Everyone doubtless has stories that parallel these. The details are rich, and the motivations on all sides are complicated. Of course the conflicts are exacerbated by restrictions in financial resources and that complex thicket of strategies for cost containment that we call managed care. I wish only to make the point that their dependence on and power over physicians is a seriously complicating factor in the life of health care organizations.

I can make this point in another way by recalling a distinction that is sometimes used in business ethics. Stockholders are persons who have made an economic investment in a firm and who hope for a financial return on their investment. Stakeholders are persons whose welfare and well-being are tied up with the fate of the firm—who have a stake in it—but who may have no investment in it in the technical economic sense of being holders of stock. Many writers in business ethics use this distinction to argue that the interests of stakeholders (e.g., employees or persons whose lives are affected by its waste products) should have some say in decisions about the firm's policies and behavior.

If we take that model, as Edward Spencer and his colleagues do,[5] as our paradigm for organizational ethics in health care, I think it will quickly become apparent that the hospital has several key stakeholders. The first and most important is certainly patients and potential patients. But close behind them is the hospital's professional staff, beginning with the physicians and nurses. These professionals should want to practice their professions at the highest possible level, and the hospital will not be able to serve patients if the professionals cannot function well. There are certainly other stakeholders—nonprofessional employees and management, the larger community, medical education programs that may be associated with the hospital—but the relationship and mutual dependency with physicians and nurses is extremely close, and one way or another these relationships must be made to work.

So the world of the hospital trustee has at least two distinctive features. One is a commitment to the pursuit of health—something we all value highly but find it difficult to define. The other is the need for cooperation or alliances with diverse constituencies in order to have a chance of attaining that goal. A modern American hospital is a classic instance of an institution of which much is expected; it is also an instance of an institution that has to play along to get along.

What Should Hospital Trustees Do?

Given this way of understanding trusteeship and hospitals, what follows for the duties of hospital trustees? No one could spell out their charge completely; the hard questions must be tackled on a case-by-case basis. But we can identify a set of general imperatives that are particularly important for hospital boards at the beginning of the twenty-first century. I want to comment on four of these imperatives: (1) the preservation of a distinctive religious identity; (2) organizational ethics; (3) the need for palliative care; and (4) a commitment to education. On all these issues, some deep-seated features of American culture are dramatically affecting the work of hospitals; on all of them it is easy to go wrong. I will take more space on some than others, assuming that what I have to say about the first two may be more controversial than my assertions about the others.

Religious Identity

In addition to the obvious historical and political reasons for careful thought about the relationship between hospitals and religious communities, there is a religious concern of great importance. In its origins, the word salvation relates to wholeness and health; saving power, in the biblical traditions from Elijah to Jesus, is manifested in physical and psychical healing. So any serious attempt to discern what it means to live a Jewish or Christian life today must relate the faith tradition to the enormous economic and psychological investment our culture has made in scientific medicine. Major religious traditions affirm the importance of medical healing, but they all set that healing in the context of a larger vision of the good life and good community. What effect should a religious affiliation have on the forms of health care provided at a hospital?

Consolidations, mergers, and acquisitions have made this a recurrent problem. In one recent case, Saint Louis University's decision to sell its hospital to Tenet Health Care Corporation, a large for-profit chain, triggered intense discussion in the American Catholic hierarchy. Church leaders were worried that the hospital would remain identifiably Catholic in name only.[6] In an example with which I am more familiar, Methodist Hospital of Indianapolis merged with University and Riley Hospitals to form Clarian Health Systems, raising concerns about loss of religious identity and mission on one side and worries about sectarianism on the other.

The issue I want to open concerns board responses to the possibility that one of the "redundancies" to be squeezed out after a merger would include dimensions of the hospital's life that were central to its religious identity. Some religious hospitals have responded to this possibility by selling themselves to a for-profit group and using the proceeds of the sale to establish a foundation that will act according to the distinctive sense of mission of the religious community or order. When a for-profit corporation acquires a nonprofit hospital, federal law and many state laws require that the hospital's assets must continue to be used for philanthropic ends. The Chronicle of Philanthropy reported in June 1997 that "more than $8.5 billion has been placed in at least 80 foundations" created in response to those laws.[7] Some of the new foundations restrict their activities to awarding grants, but others undertake fund-raising, which may support indigent care and other services eliminated by the hospital's new owner.

The full effectiveness of this strategy remains to be seen, but we can understand why it is not always adopted. Once the organic connection is severed, even a large foundation may find that its influence is diminished. So, many religious communities elect to sustain the identification of their religious community with a hospital. There are several ways in which a hospital might be religious, or what religious affiliation might mean.

Saying a hospital is religious may tell us something about the personnel involved, that is, about the patients or perhaps the staff. The hospital may see its role primarily as service to members of the sponsoring religious community. There is no doubt about the importance of this factor in the founding of religiously sponsored hospitals in the nineteenth and early twentieth centuries. Nor is it trivial. Insofar as religion shapes a view of the world, we might expect some increase in value agreements among adherents of any one religious tradition, at least agreement about forms of religion they reject.

However, there are practical difficulties in maintaining a hospital's religious identity in this sense, at least in a highly mobile society. Furthermore, acceptance of federal funding—a necessity for any modern American hospital—means that the hospital cannot restrict its services to members of any one religious community—if indeed any ever hoped to do that. As a practical matter, few hospitals are religious in this demographic sense.

Saying that a hospital is religious may mean that worship is conducted on its premises. The hospital might sponsor, facilitate, or simply tolerate forms of devotion. In this sense, most American hospitals are religious, as few, if any, of them prohibit all acts of worship. To be sure, the hospital may impose de facto restrictions on what worship may be done; animal sacrifice may be prohibited. But on the whole, American hospitals are very tolerant of diverse expressions of religious devotion. One would not need to worry that one would be forbidden to pray or receive the Eucharist after a merger. Mass is regularly said in Catholic hospitals, but not only in Catholic hospitals.

A hospital might be said to be religious if it offers pastoral services provided by chaplains. That is a heavier religious involvement in the sense that the religious personnel are paid by the hospital, but the exclusive linkage with a particular community is characteristically broken. Some chaplains on the payroll are identified with a particular religious community; others are not. On the whole, chaplaincy is a clerical role cut loose from specific denominational or faith–tradition ties. Thus provision of chaplaincy services might make a hospital religious in a general sense; it would not make a hospital Jewish, Catholic, or Presbyterian unless there were something exclusively Jewish, Catholic, or Presbyterian about the staff or the services it provides.

A hospital might be said to be religious in virtue of ongoing economic ties to a sponsoring religious body. Certainly many religiously affiliated hospitals began with resources provided by religious communities. Now, however, denominational support accounts for only a small fraction of hospital revenues. Need for the religious community's financial support is seldom an issue in merger discussions.

Politically, a hospital might be said to be religious if a given religious community plays a crucial role in its governance. Issues of degree may be important here. For example, the denomination's role in governance may be limited to the judicatory head's ex officio seat on the board; the situation would be different if the denomination had greater power to determine board membership or key administrative appointments. Still, maintaining a role in governance is a significant form of religiousness or identification with the sponsoring religious community. Of course, the larger issue is "to what end is this power held?"

Finally, we would say that a hospital is morally religious, if care and services provided by the hospital cohere with the key views and values of the sponsoring religious community. In some cases, this coherence may be obvious, as some services, such as abortions or sterilizations, are simply not provided. But restricting patient services to be provided is only one dimension of the hospital's life that a religious community might affect. For example, religious values can be components of a corporate culture, and sustaining those values is an important component in preserving religious identity.

Among these options, the pastoral, political, and moral components of ongoing religious identity should be of greatest concern to trustees. On a pastoral level, recollection of the founding vision suggests that pastoral needs must be attended to, even if those needs are not always seen to be just what the founders saw them to be. For example, awareness of increased and more articulate cultural pluralism is a fact of American life that must be acknowledged by commitment to the common good and social justice. So a religious sponsor should want to ensure that provision of high-quality pastoral care (not excluding appropriate worship opportunities) will be an important feature of the life of the new entity. This in effect requires an interfaith chaplaincy service that is competent and adequately budgeted as part of the legacy of the founders.

The moral stance of the community also should have an ongoing legacy, but that is a harder issue because morality necessarily faces outward toward others. Many religious communities that have sponsored hospitals in the United States—I immediately think of Judaism, Catholicism, and Methodism—have strong, religiously based commitments to social justice and serving poor people. It is hard to imagine a religiously identified hospital that holds those commitments agreeing to a merger or reformulation of identity that would allow those commitments to be diluted.

But one reason this point seems obvious is that there is convergence between the religious traditions and a common morality of social justice. That convergence does not exist across the range of moral issues on which religious communities have taken stands—issues as diverse as the legitimacy of autopsy, abortion, use of alcoholic beverages, in vitro fertilization, or physician-assisted suicide. Here there will be many hard cases and good faith disagreements about how closely a merged entity must hew to the line of the founding tradition in order rightly to be called Jewish, Catholic, or Methodist.

It would be foolish to attempt to answer this question in the abstract, but I think it reasonable to assert that this is a case where the extreme positions are clearly wrong. On the one hand, it is unreasonable to suggest that no religiously particular practices may be sustained. Public morality does not require exact uniformity of service provision across differing hospitals anymore than it is wrong for publicly funded schools to have distinctive identities and profiles. On the other hand, religious communities must be willing to acknowledge that some of their moral commitments have a stronger foundation in common morality than others. For example, and without offering my own comment on the merits of either issue, the Roman Catholic opposition to abortion has a stronger foundation in common morality than the tradition's opposition to voluntary sterilization. It should be easier for a Catholic hospital to give up a prohibition on sterilization than one on abortion, if the board takes seriously its commitment to social justice and the common good.

Concern for the political identification of the hospital with a religious community should not be important for its own sake, but as a way of ensuring the vitality of the pastoral and moral components. Judicatory heads or their appointees (or both) may find it important to have seats on the board to assure that commitments to pastoral care and moral medical practice are sustained. This presence may diminish to the purest tokenism, and religiously identified board members will need to hone their skills and be assured that governance procedures will give them a fair hearing.

Contemporary American society will not make discussions about religious communities' distinctive moral views easy. On both the religious and secular sides of the argument, we have a tendency to equate religion with the irrational and then either reject it for that reason or favor an intellectual leap in which we take a great deal on faith. The idea that religion in general, and religiously based morality in particular, is something that can and should be reasoned about does not come easily to many Americans. But hospital boards should model reasoned discussion and come to the best accommodations they can in their particular times and places.

Organizational Ethics

Trustees committed to a fidelity principle and to the common good will want to assure the highest levels of professionalism and ethical practice in the hospital. Getting that assurance requires moves in two different directions, and to explain that I need to quickly summarize a couple of ideas of the Protestant theologian Reinhold Niebuhr. Niebuhr was preoccupied with the problem of power—with reconciliation of an ethics of love with the responsible use of force or coercion.

The key insight in Niebuhr's reconciliation of love and the use of force was an analysis of human selfhood. He defined the human being as a "finite spirit." As "spirits" we are conscious beings, but we are aware of our finitude; we know that we will die, and the result is that our lives are characterized by fear or—as the existentialists used to say—anxiety. The combination of freedom and finitude for a self-transcendent being is terrifying. Niebuhr generalized the kinds of responses people make to anxiety into two broad types. Each shows the effects of anxiety on our relations with others. On the one hand, we may manifest the "will to live truly" or love—an altruistic commitment to serve others. More typically, however, people respond to anxiety in destructive ways. Some retreat from the terror of freedom and deny their self-transcendence by trying to forget it or blot out anxiety in substance abuse or sensuality. More typically, persons ignore their finitude and pretend that their ideas, hopes, and plans are of infinite worth; that we are not finite and limited. That is pride.

The usual symptom of pride is a desire to do better than other persons, seeing human relations in comparative and competitive terms. I not only want a good salary; I want a better salary than Bill Brightguy, who just published a book that was favorably reviewed in the *New York Times*. Consciousness after the Fall, as the theologians might put it, is inevitably comparative, competitive, and relational. Thus Niebuhr thought that persons have a possibility of acting cooperatively, in love. But this kind of action, redeemed from terror, was difficult to attain and not to be counted on. This analysis led Niebuhr to his oft-quoted aphorism: "Man's capacity for justice makes democracy possible; man's capacity for injustice makes democracy necessary."

Above, I noted the importance of the relationship between health professionals and hospitals. If we think about this relationship with Niebuhr's analysis in the back of our minds, two conclusions will be apparent. The first is that even the most well-intentioned professionals must be under some pressure to do the right thing. Good will is not enough. So part of the mechanism of organizational ethics in a hospital must involve having effective procedures for credentialing, one or more effective clinical ethics committees, and in many settings an IRB. Procedures for review and discipline of physicians, nurses, administrators, and other professionals and staff must be in place.

Good organizational ethics also requires creating possibilities of mutual help and support. It requires effective dialogic relations with major professional groups, notably physicians and nurses. The word dialogic is crucial here. Dialogue is precisely not a situation in which one's only objective is to persuade the person or persons with whom one is speaking. Effective representation, even attempts at persuasion, are important components in dialogue, but they are only part of the story. For dialogue implies listening. We do not have dialogue if the concerned parties are unwilling to listen, learn, and change their positions. That is not to say that no one can ever hold fast in dialogue. Sometimes I *am* right. But it is to say that I must be and appear to be open to receipt of new information. The dialogic process must make those facts apparent.

Effective organizational ethics for hospitals today requires the creation of space—perhaps neutral space—in which administrators and physicians can talk together about their visions for the hospital and the difficulties of professional practice. Although it may be most efficient for these to be discussions in the board room or between the chief of the medical staff and the chief executive officer, the effect will be much better and communication more thorough if the conversations are going in multiple and perhaps deescalated venues. Effective dialogue is not always efficient; indeed, it is time consuming. But it is essential to the good functioning of a health care institution.

The imperative for dialogue is particularly important with nursing, a profession caught in the middle, invaluable yet vulnerable. Nurses must have more real power in health care organizations than they now have. Although there is a proud history of persons moving from nursing into the highest ranks of hospital administration, nurses on the floors often feel disenfranchised and powerless. Something has to happen to change that.

Palliation

Third, a concern with founding mission and the common good requires hospitals to be committed to palliative care. As is well known, the demographics and circumstances of dying have changed in the past century. Whereas 100 years ago most people died from accidents or infection, today we die from malignancies and cardiovascular problems. We die older, after a lengthy period of decline, and often separated from family and home. Dying has gotten worse, thanks to the wonderful century of medical progress from which we have all benefited.

These "modern" deaths are too often accompanied by pain, shortness of breath, dementia, delirium, nausea, and constipation. Palliative care is the medical field that addresses these issues. It is closely related to the hospice movement. Taking palliative care seriously means two things for a hospital.

First, it means acknowledging the reality of death as compatible with health. Death is the normal and appropriate end of a healthy life. No adequate definition of health as the goal of health care can ignore this fact. Of course, death may be untimely, and people usually come to hospitals hoping and expecting to be cured. But it requires an intolerable act of institutional denial to pretend that people do not die in hospitals, or that attention to their distinctive needs near the end of life is somehow not part of the hospital's mandate. I concede that provision of fine end of life care may not be the easiest achievement for a hospital to use to market itself, but in fact having that kind of reputation will greatly enhance the institution's stature in the community.

Preparing itself to deliver quality palliative care requires a hospital to do some resource allocation or reallocation as well as to be honest with itself. Palliative care begins with effective pain management, and learning how to do that—as well as how to manage other discomforts near the end of life—is a significant technical skill like surgery or anesthesiology. Palliative care specialists should be as important to a medical staff as cardiologists. Further, palliative care requires attention to many social, psychological, religious or spiritual, and even economic issues. It is unrealistic—and undesirable—to expect most hospitals to be able to adequately address this range of issues using their own resources and staffs. But they have to be able to make connections and to assure themselves that crucial needs are met.

Education

Sustaining religious identity requires serious thought about religion; dialogue with professionals requires an investment of time and a capacity for understanding; learning how to care for the dying requires the recognition of problems and the development of skills. None of these objectives can be achieved without a serious investment in education—education of professionals, hospital staff and administration, and the larger community.

William F. May, another contributor to this volume, has argued strongly for the centrality of teaching to the physician's role. He argues that doctors should acknowledge their indebtedness to society as a whole, and that this acknowledgment transforms the physician's relationship to patients. It does not mean that physicians lose authority, but that they have the kind of authority of a teacher rather than of a military commander who gives "orders." Effective health care entails a partnership between physicians and patients, an engagement with patients as persons.[8]

Hospitals stand to society as a whole as physicians stand to their patients. They have a comparable responsibility to take a leadership role in discussion of serious issues relating to health care. I have just tried to specify three key issues that should be on this educational agenda: the fact of the inevitability of death and the importance of palliative care, the relationship between religion and medicine, and the importance and limits of professional autonomy. A hospital betrays its trust if it fails to step outside the crucial terrain of provision of services to enter the realm of public conversation.

American hospitals early in the twenty-first century should look different from each other. But they should have some things in common. A key role of their trustees is assuring their moral integrity, i.e., their fidelity to their historic mission, their service to the common good, and their fair dealing with the members of their communities. We can say further that moral integrity in this time and place requires investing in pastoral care services and palliative care and engaging in the time-consuming tasks of professional, patient, and public education. These are moral imperatives that cannot be ignored.

Notes

1. David H. Smith, *Entrusted: The Moral Responsibilities of Trusteeship*, ed. Robert L. Payton and Dwight Burlingame, Philanthropic Studies (Bloomington: Indiana University Press, 1995).

2. Norman Daniels, *Just Health Care* (Cambridge: Cambridge University Press, 1988), 23.

3. Daniels, *Just Health Care*. See also Leon R. Kass, *Toward a More Natural Science: Biology and Human Affairs* (New York: Free Press, 1985), 157–86.

4. Daniel F. Chambliss, *Beyond Caring: Hospitals, Nurses and the Social Organization of Ethics* (Chicago: University of Chicago Press, 1996).

5. Edward M. Spencer, Ann E. Mills, Mary V. Rorty, and Patricia H. Werhane, eds., *Organization Ethics in Health Care* (New York: Oxford University Press, 2000).

6. John F. Kavenaugh, "Capitalism's Cost to Care," *America* 178, no. 8 (March 14, 1998): 37; Pamela Schaffer, "Cardinals Claim Rights in Hospital Dispute," *National Catholic Reporter*, October 24, 1997, 3.

7. Jon Craig and Holly Hall, "For-Sale Signs at Hospitals Chill Giving," *Chronicle of Philanthropy*, June 12, 1997, 1.

8. William F. May, *The Physician's Covenant: Images of the Healer in Medical Ethics* (Philadelphia: Westminster Press, 1983).

8

TRUSTEESHIP AS REPRESENTATION

Bruce Jennings

A useful distinction in thinking about the ethics of hospital trustees is that between the "ethics of trusteeship" and "ethics in trusteeship." The ethics *of* trusteeship is the study of the general ethical obligations and permissions that are constitutive of the role or office of trustee as such. Ethics *in* trusteeship pertains to the day-to-day ethical quandaries that arise in the practice of being a trustee and in the decisions trustees must make.

In this chapter, my focus will be primarily on the ethics of trusteeship. In particular, I ask to what extent it is illuminating to see trusteeship as a kind of representation, as fulfilling a type of representative function, and as occupying a niche in a larger overall structure of political and ethical representation in American society.

THE REPRESENTATIONAL SOCIETY

There can be no doubt that we have become, through practical necessity, a society of representation through and through. After all, a system of representation is integral to a legitimate constitutional democracy. But representation is not limited to the government or the political realm. There are several domains of what might loosely and generically be called "unelected representation."[1] The arena of professional practice is one such domain. Ours is a society made up of complex, interdependent, and often conflicting interests, and a society increasingly dependent on expertise; so many specialized functions and authority are delegated to individuals designated as "professionals," who are charged with representing, in some sense, the interests of clients, institutions, organizations, and society at large.

Another important domain of unelected representation is the press—the print and broadcast news media. It is appropriate to capture this form of representation under the heading of professional activity and professional ethics, because journalism is properly seen as a profession in its own right, and in some sense readers and viewers are the "clients" of this profession to whom various duties are owed. However, the news media seem also to transcend the scope of other professions because they have become the closest thing we seem to have in contemporary society to a common culture and an authoritative record of opinions and events.[2] As our common link, however, the news media play a crucial role in representing reality to a mass audience; and in exercising their news judgments about what to select for scarce print space or air time, journalists have an obligation to represent the interests of their readers and viewers. Many decisions in private life are made on the basis of information conveyed by the media, and, although it now seems quaint, the long-standing observation that the press is the necessary foundation of democratic citizenship remains true. The unelected representation performed by journalists makes the elected representation of our governmental system possible.

Finally, a very important domain of unelected representation takes place within what is generally known as "civil society": the sphere of voluntary, mediating institutions that stand between the individual and the state. The domain of civil society is also frequently differentiated from the realm of competitive, profit-oriented economic activity known as the market. In civil society, voluntary associations, clubs, groups, faith-based bodies including churches, and nonprofit organizations all have in some sense a public interest and public service orientation. Although the organizations of civil society normally encourage direct participation and activity by their members on the local, and sometimes the state and national levels as well, direct participation by large numbers of rank-and-file members of any organization is the exception rather than the rule and is normally not practical except in the most extraordinary circumstances. So representation is one of the key activities of the institutions of civil society inasmuch as they serve to advocate on behalf of their members or on behalf of those who are not adequately served by the established modes of electoral, political, and governmental representation. The leadership of civil society organizations, including paid staff, activist members, and members of their governing boards, form a level of unelected representation that is becoming increasingly important in contemporary society.

It is here, of course, that the not-for-profit hospital and its leadership enter the domain of unelected representation. Thus far, I have been using the term "unelected" in a broad and informal sense to designate the world of nongovernmental organizations, outside the structure of constitutional political representation (in Congress; state legislatures; and county, city, and town councils) and outside the formal mechanisms of electoral selection of official representatives. With hospital trustees, however, the term is more precise and accurate. Many civil society organizations have some electoral or quasi-electoral mechanisms as a part of their bylaws and operating procedures. Hospital boards tend on the whole to be self-perpetuating in the sense that the boards themselves determine the bylaws, control the nominating process, and select their own members.

With a hospital board of trustees, there is literally no opportunity for an individual to be selected who is somehow officially or electorally beholden to a particular constituency or set of hospital stakeholders, unless perhaps it is a subgroup of the existing trustees and management who sponsored and supported his or her selection to the board. Most commonly, however, no such ties are made explicit; it goes against the subtle cultural styles and traditions operative on not-for-profit boards in most places.

Thus a new hospital trustee literally assumes his or her office in a vacuum—owing favors to no one, oriented toward no particular set of interests or beliefs save those growing out of the trustee's own personal experience or background. Personal conflicts of interest aside, this is in a sense the ideal situation one wants for a trustee because this lack of ties and obligations may permit the individual to take a genuinely objective orientation toward the mission of the institution, its best interests, the best interests of the hospital's stakeholders, and the common good of the community as a whole. Conversely, there is a parallel danger implicit in this free-floating, representationally nonresponsible posture, and that is the possibility that such an individual will be an easy target for the persuasion and manipulation of particular factions or interest groups within the hospital or outside it. Lacking ties, the trustee also may lack concern and commitment. Lacking obligations and promises to keep, the trustee may also lack any sense of purpose.

From the point of view of the notion of representation and its various social functions, then, the not-for-profit hospital trustee is in an awkward position. On the one hand, he or she seemingly stands outside the domain of representation altogether, but on the other hand the need to represent and give voice to certain groups and perspectives is a necessity that virtually every trustee feels at one time or another.

Just whom or what is the trustee supposed to represent? Of course, trustees are responsible for the welfare of the hospital, and in some attenuated sense they may be said to represent the hospital's interests. As the present author and his colleagues make clear in their essay "Ethics and Trusteeship for Healthcare: Hospital Board Service in Turbulent Times," this viewpoint carries with it some serious ethical problems and is at best a partial statement of the actual basis and scope of a trustee's responsibilities.[3] For my purposes here, this response is incomplete and unsatisfactory because it begs the question. To what individuals and to what specific interests and values should the trustee give voice in the deliberations of the board and in his or her other activities as a trustee? There are no formal laws or mechanisms of accountability that will pressure a given trustee to play the role of representative in this sense. The impulse to do so comes almost entirely from the conscience and awareness of the trustee himself or herself—an awareness that representation on behalf of someone and something is needed.

One other notion of "representation" frequently arises in the context of civic organizations such as hospitals, particularly those that have some identification with communities marked by high degrees of ethnic and racial diversity. This is the idea that a board can be representative of the community it serves if it has the same or similar ethnic composition as that community. The corollary of this notion at the level of the individual trustee is that having a trustee of the same ethnic or racial background as the community in question automatically makes that individual a representative of that group.

There are numerous problems with this identity concept of representation. It certainly does not follow that an African American trustee, for example, will automatically be a representative of the African American community surrounding the hospital. For one thing, considerations of class and gender complicate this relationship considerably. Moreover, it tends to point the attention of the representative in the wrong direction by suggesting that the representational skills and capacities of the trustee lie within, in his or her own racial and ethnic experiences growing up in a context of discrimination and inequality, rather than consisting in the ability and willingness of the representative to turn outward to the constituency in question in order to listen to and learn from them. In my view, the skills of representation lie more with those outward orientations than with the personal experiences of the individual. Perhaps having the same traditions or racial characteristics as a particular group does assist the person to communicate and empathize with other members of that group. But it is also true that members of a minority group who succeed in achieving upward social mobility during the course of their lifetimes are often more critical and less sympathetic to their racial or ethnic peers who have been left behind than are those coming from a significantly different personal experience and whose empathy and sympathy are sustained by moral convictions and a sense of justice.

Arguments of this kind do not show that trustees should never be selected because they, in their very persons, add ethnic, racial, or gender diversity to a board. There are times when doing so is wise and has salutatory effects. It increases a sense of pride and dignity in the affected community. It may lend an important new tone and dynamic to interpersonal relations on the board. It may make an important symbolic statement by the hospital to the community and help to restore trust. However, I do question the notion that having the composition of the board mirror the composition of the surrounding community ipso facto makes the board more representative or, to put the point more precisely, a more effective and ethical representational institution. In fact, representation is an exceedingly complex concept and practice.

In the light of these considerations, it is not surprising that Bradford Gray and Linda Weiss found that many of the trustees they interviewed were prone to link their perception of ethical issues faced by trustees with the question of how the trustee should serve as a representative of a voiceless or powerless group on a board generally composed of the affluent and the well connected (see chapter 5 in the present volume).

THE CONCEPT OF REPRESENTATION

To represent is to make present something that is literally physically absent here and now. Thus, a painting or photograph may represent a person who is far away or no longer living. It may even represent an imaginary person who exists only in the mind of the painter. Language and other semiotic systems have the capacity to represent ideas or objects in the same way. Applied to human interactions, this capacity to make the literally absent symbolically present makes possible a whole range of transactions that could not be undertaken if the physical presence of all parties were required.[4]

For centuries, political theorists have recognized that the institution of representation holds the key to governance that is both practical and morally legitimate, particularly from a democratic point of view. Governance by the direct participation of all the affected parties is normally impossible, undesirable, or both. It is impossible because direct participatory assemblies—ancient Athens, the Swiss canton, the New England town meeting—are workable only on a very small scale. Moreover, plebiscite arrangements, which permit direct participation of large numbers of impersonal citizens, are undesirable because they reflect choices and judgments made on the basis of tainted and one-sided information and uninformed by the process of face-to-face deliberation and debate that is possible in small direct assemblies or in larger representational ones. Therefore, under the conditions of the modern nation-state, the institution of representation allows for governance *of* all the people but *by* only a few of the people.[5]

Within various accounts of representation, two basic pairs of concepts have been dominant. The first pair consists of the notion of "direct" and "virtual" representation. These notions are not crucial to the present discussion. Direct representation insists that the person who will perform the representation be chosen by those whom he or she represents. Virtual representation allows for more informal, self-appointed representatives, such as the unelected representation I have been discussing in connection with the role of hospital trustee.

The second pair of concepts, however, is more important for our purposes. It refers to how a representative should go about representing, not how he or she should be selected. One is the "delegate" conception of representation. According to this view, the representative has an obligation to convey only the messages, opinions, and positions of those represented, and should serve as the advocate for these positions in the legislative or governing process.

The other traditional view, interestingly enough, is called the "trustee" conception of representation. This trustee conception, made famous in the writings of the eighteenth-century British political theorist and politician Edmund Burke, holds that the represented has no obligation to convey only the particular opinions and views of his or her constituents. What the representative owes those represented instead is his or her best thinking and judgment about what would be in the best interest of the represented, whether they currently view matters that way or not.

Neither of these one-dimensional conceptions of representation is really adequate, and the actual practice of representation tends to be a balance and combination of the delegate and the trustee functions, a balance between making the actual interests and preferences of the constituents present in the legislative process and making and more paternalistically promoting those interests that the representative thinks would be the best for those represented.

The same balance must be struck by hospital trustees as they perform a representative function in hospital governance. Hospital trustees must not act only as "trustees" but also as delegates to some extent. This is made all the more difficult because the hospital trustee may not in the nature of the case have regular links or direct lines of communication with the individuals or groups that he or she wishes to serve. So the question arises of how the trustee is to be a delegate if he or she does not know what messages to carry, what positions and preferences to represent. The answer is that if the hospital trustee is going to attempt to play the role of representative at all, such lines of communication must be opened up.

This conveys a real advantage for the trustee style of representation as well, for it also presupposes a close communication and working knowledge of the lives and experiences of the outside group. How else is the trustee to make judgments about the best interests of others? The trustee-style representative can no more afford to be aloof and disconnected from the constituency in question than can a delegate-style representative.

Legitimate democratic representation requires that representatives embody three important moral or civic virtues. Representatives should be morally independent agents whose decisions are based on rational, informed, unbiased, and uncoerced judgments. Representatives should be accountable and responsive to constituents' interests, while at the same time informing and educating constituents about what reasonably can be accomplished. And finally, representatives should act in ways that help sustain or improve systems of governance and decision making that are responsive to the legitimate interests of all citizens and to the common good of the nation as a whole.

The ethical duties that logically stem from these fundamental requirements of legitimate democratic representation are based on what I shall call the principles of independence, accountability, and responsibility. These principles constitute the generic framework for the ethics of representation.[6] They define the basic obligations of all those who play a significant role in the representational process, and therefore they apply to elected and unelected representatives alike, including not-for-profit hospital trustees. In what follows, I offer a framework for the analysis of the ethics of representation by discussing these three principles, and I attempt to draw out some of the implications of these principles for the practice of hospital trusteeship.

THE ETHICS OF REPRESENTATION

When an individual steps into the role of representative, he or she takes on a second ethical identity, one composed of a structure of special obligations that are often more demanding and restrictive than the general moral obligations of private life. To assume the role of representative is to make a special promise to the rest of us, and to accept a special trust on our behalf. These obligations are obviously most binding when one has become a representative as a result of a formal electoral process, but they have ethical force even when the representation is virtual and the representative is self-appointed.

What, precisely, is the content of that trust? Answering this question takes us to the heart of what we mean by representation in a democracy and in a democratic culture, in which persons significantly affected by decisions made by those in a position of power have a right to some say or influence in the making of those decisions. When it comes to hospital governance, patients and their families, the professional and support staff, and the surrounding community as a whole all certainly are affected in ways that bring them routinely within this ambit of democratic accountability. As I understand them, the principles of representational ethics derive from our nation's democratic traditions and from our understanding of the political conditions necessary to sustain the legitimacy and health of the democratic way of life. The ethical duties of representatives that follow from these fundamental requirements of legitimate democratic representation are based on the principles of independence, accountability, and responsibility.

Independence

The principle of independence holds that representatives have an obligation to deliberate and decide, free from improper influence. In making policy, it is impossible to ensure that all decisions that representatives make will be wise ones. Representatives, like all other human beings, make mistakes, commit errors of fact and judgment, and have imperfect foresight into the consequences of their actions. But by taking steps to preserve the independence of their judgments, they can at least increase the probability that they will judge and decide correctly.

The idea behind the principle of independence is the assumption that representational decision making is less likely to be intelligent and fair if representatives make decisions in an atmosphere of improper influence. The problem raised by the application of this principle in specific situations is to determine what counts as improper influence.

A representative's duty to act independently and to avoid factors that compromise independence does not mean that he or she should be isolated from all influences or should try to make decisions in some kind of vacuum. Isolating representatives from all influences would be both unworkable and unacceptable. Properly functioning institutions of representation clearly require that representatives remain open to many kinds of outside influence, and that they remain accessible and responsive to both constituent interest and the public interest.

How then to draw the line between proper and improper influences? Improper influences are ones that tend to distract representatives from their basic functions. They draw representatives' use of the authority and resources of their position away from the public ends—the representation of constituent interest and the promotion of the public interest—that these positions were created to serve in the first place.

To preserve their independence, hospital trustees as representatives must avoid becoming too dependent on any single source of information or analysis. In their careers and other community activities, trustees necessarily form close associations with local businesspeople, advocates, special interest groups, and others who have a distinct stake in the way hospitals operate. But these special associations must not become the exclusive source of a trustee's perspective and outlook; their influence becomes improper when they come to distract the trustee from his or her broader ethical responsibilities to patients, health professionals, the surrounding community, and the hospital and board as institutions. Trustees who, in the overall pattern of the roles they play, become simply the spokespeople for the narrow interests and objectives of specially favored groups violate the principle of independence as seriously as those who attempt to steer hospital contracts or other favors to vendors in return for financial benefits.

Accountability

The principle of accountability holds that representatives have an obligation to provide constituents with the information and understanding those constituents require to exercise responsible democratic citizenship or to attend to their civic and personal interests in a properly informed and effective way. Because representatives have wide discretion in their activities, and because no theory of representation or representational ethics can prescribe all the choices they must make, the ultimate check against improper representational conduct and the ultimate support for proper representational conduct must come from either constituents, peers, or a higher legal authority. This is the core of the traditional democratic idea that the authority of those who govern rests on the consent of those who are governed—albeit that in many cases the consent is indirect. The idea behind the principle of accountability is that representatives themselves ought to take reasonable steps to ensure that democratic consent is fully informed and enlightened.

In the case of hospital trustees on self-perpetuating boards, stakeholders or constituents have no direct mechanism either to select or to remove a trustee; hence, that task falls to the other members of the board and, in extreme cases, to the attorney general of the state within which the hospital is incorporated or the state courts. Nonetheless, the evaluation and response by stakeholders concerning a trustee's performance can be—and, I would argue, should be—one important factor in determining the response of peers or higher authorities.

The fact of the matter is, however, that this sort of check on accountability rarely comes into play. Stakeholders do not have the necessary information to evaluate a trustee's performance in light of their interests and values when minutes and other public documentation of board activity are vague and nonspecific concerning the comments or votes of particular board members. More commonly, stakeholders react to large decisions made by the board as a whole and evaluate the board en masse. This type of single-issue evaluation and generalization is hardly ideal and can be quite unfair to individual trustees. But it seems unlikely that strong mechanisms of democratic accountability are going to be imported into the customary world of hospital trusteeship any time soon. That leaves accountability mainly in the hands of the other trustees who are in a position to see how a person has argued, voted, and behaved during their term of office. The board chair may be in the best position of all to make such evaluations, with the advice of senior hospital management.

The problems of applying the principle of accountability arise in determining what kinds of information are integral to the constituents' exercise of responsible democratic citizenship or reasonable decision making in personal life. Where do we draw the line between what those represented need to know and do not need to know?

The duty of accountability involves many aspects of a representative's activities. Constituents need to be able to monitor representational activities so that they can provide feedback to representatives concerning needs and interests that have been neglected. If hospital trustees were to operate in a more representative fashion, records of decision making and hospital operations would have to be more openly disclosed. Even with such things as medical error and patient safety concerns, that kind of public or community accountability has been very controversial. Unlike government officials, hospitals and trustees are not protected in various ways from civil lawsuits. When a response at the ballot box on election day is not an option, recourse to lawsuits is the companion of the principle of accountability. Here, admittedly, adhering to ethical standards requires courage and a willingness to defend one's actions and record if necessary.

Accountability is not simply a burden imposed on representatives by a long democratic tradition that has always been wary of anyone holding a position of political power. It also has a more positive and constructive rationale. When it gives citizens the information and understanding they need to become more thoughtful partners in the process of representation, accountability enables representatives to be more effective. They can provide intellectual and political leadership on important issues, and at the same time they can benefit and learn from their constituents.

Moreover, remaining accountable in this sense helps representatives fulfill their duty to be open-minded, independent decision makers. This may seem like a paradox, but it is not. The principle of accountability does not require that a representative keep a constant eye on the polls and bend to each passing political wind. On the contrary. Accountability reinforces a balanced representational style—part delegate who should conscientiously convey to the board the preferences of the represented, and part trustee-leader who should work to educate the represented and to change those preferences if they are misguided. Maintaining a well-informed, alert constituency is one of the representative's best protections against falling into an ethically dangerous dependence on narrow or biased advice, from whatever source.

Finally, citizens need more than factual information; they need a context within which to interpret the significance of the information they receive about representatives. Accountability requires representatives not only to disclose what they have done but also to explain and justify it.

Responsibility

The principle of responsibility holds that representatives have an obligation to contribute to the effective institutional functioning of the representational process. Representation and governance are collective processes; they rely on the cooperation and coordinated activities of many participants in an overall system. For example, individual trustees cannot fulfill the ethical obligations of their office or role merely by attending to their own activities and their own pet projects. They must be concerned as well with the activities of other trustees and with the functioning of the board and the hospital as a whole.

The problems of applying the principle of responsibility arise in determining what the "effective institutional functioning" of representational institutions requires. To be responsible, hospital trustees must strike a delicate balance between accommodating themselves to the existing institutional and procedural arrangements of their board or hospital and pressing for organizational change through internal, private criticism, public statements, and institutional leadership. The principle of responsibility does not charge trustees with an obligation to accept uncritically the institutional status quo. But it does require that they direct their efforts to bring about institutional reform in ways that will enhance the service orientation and the representative functions of hospital governance and management.

TRUSTEESHIP AS REPRESENTATION

Having outlined a generic framework for the ethics of representation, let me now attempt to spell out in more detail how these ethical principles might apply to hospital trustee decision-making and practices.

The principle of independence suggests that trustees should make hospital policy and chief executive officer personnel decisions free from improper influences. Trustees must strive to remain open-minded, and adequately and independently informed. They must avoid placing themselves or being placed in situations that would compromise their independent judgment through coercion, bias, or conflict of interest. The principle of independence is thus closely related to the need for trustees to have access to reliable information and objective data, and to make decisions based on this objective information. In the past, too many boards have not been supplied in a timely and complete manor with objective information concerning hospital finances and budgeting or financial and business plans associated with capital improvement projects or service delivery ventures.

The principle of independence also suggests a much less passive and reactive image of the trustee as an ethical actor and decision maker than one finds in descriptions of trustee behavior in the academic literature (cf. chapter 3 in this volume). Trustees do not and should not simply react to seemingly neutral information or facts with which they are presented. All sources of information require active interpretation and judgment. This does not mean that there is no distinction to be drawn between reasonable and unreasonable decisions, or well-informed versus biased and cavalier judgments. But it does mean that trustee decision making involves all the characteristic ingredients of human judgment—discernment, selectivity, setting priorities, and balancing conflicting values—and as such is subject to a broad range of influences.

Independence requires open-mindedness, listening carefully to all sides and reflecting on them. In the course of their work and life in a given neighborhood or community, trustees necessarily form associations with people who have special interest and axes to grind. Independence means not being dependent on a single source of information and not allowing the value of the source of information to turn into an obligation to that source. It means separating professional and personal relationships, so that the interests of the latter do not undermine the responsibilities of the former. And it means remaining insulated from the business or economic interests of the many vendors and outside organizations that do significant business with the hospital or indeed come into competition with it.

As the trend toward physician group practice and setting up physician-controlled diagnostic centers or outpatient clinics continues, the service on hospital boards by influential physicians in the community who are tied to these practices but also enjoy hospital privileges becomes problematic, to say the least. The same may be true of trustees who are local business owners for whom the hospital, or health care programs closely related to the hospital, may be potential clients or customers.

Recusal from participation and voting on a particular matter before the board is often the best means to handle such conflicts of interest and compromises of independence. Resignation or the decision to forgo board service altogether is more drastic but may sometimes be necessary. By the same token, conflict of interest can be seen as a matter of degree. From a representational point of view, it is an advantage to have a physician on the board and to have local businesspeople, as well as labor leaders, clergy, neighborhood leaders, and the like. It would be counterproductive if the ethics of hospital trusteeship were understood to preclude board service by such persons. In some small, closely knit communities, the thicket of at least potential conflict of interest is so dense that eliminating it entirely would virtually mean that no one but detached commuters could serve on the board.

The principle of accountability suggests that trustees have an obligation to use the resources of the hospital to provide patients, staff, and community members with the information and understanding they require to make decisions about health care in their own best interests and in the public interest. Hospitals are often seen only as venues of emergency and acute care; in fact, they are often centers for public health, health promotion and maintenance, preventive medicine, and public health education and health literacy in their communities. These are no less important or worthy of a trustee's time and attention than the quality standards of the emergency room or the intensive care unit. What I am suggesting is that the principle of accountability be understood on two levels for trustees. The first level has to do with monitoring and evaluating the performance of the trustee during his or her term of office. The second level has to do with the trustee's role, via the hospital, in educating and empowering stakeholders to improve their own decisions and to take more control of the conditions of their own lives.

What makes a trustee accountable? Part of this involves disclosure of financial interests, of entangling personal relationships, of an attitudinal bias one way or the other toward individuals, groups, or public policies. Another reinforcement of accountability comes from access. Trustees should make themselves available to talk with community members, patients and families, and hospital staff. Hospitals should be open about their governance policies, standards, and procedures.

The basic question for accountability, as I am using the concept here, is: What do citizens need to know to assess, evaluate, and use the information they are getting from the health care system? If we ideally expect hospitals not merely to treat disease but also to inform and to educate about health, there is no good reason why we ought not expect the same of hospital trustees.

Finally, the principle of responsibility suggests that trustees have an obligation to contribute to the effective institutional functioning of boards and hospitals so as to make their role in the overall process of representation independent and accountable. Like individual legislators who serve in legislative institutions and must be responsible participants in a collective legislative process, and like congressional candidates who should be responsible participants in a democratic electoral process that does not exist simply to serve their own political self-interest and ambition, unelected representatives such as individual trustees also have ethical obligations as members of boards and as participants in a collective process of hospital governance.

The principle of responsibility calls attention to the fact that any individual trustee's ability to perform his or her role ethically is at least partially dependent on the conduct of other trustees and the ethical ethos or climate that is established within hospital boards and the corporate culture of the hospital as a whole. Conscientious trustees have an interest in helping to maintain an organizational ethos that supports independent and accountable trustee decision making and governance; they also have an obligation to contribute to that ethos or to help create it when it does not exist. Although the burden of this responsibility falls on all trustees and hospital managers, it is especially significant for board chairs, committee chairs, experienced trustees, top hospital executives, and senior leaders on the medical and nursing staffs who are in a position to influence policy and serve as ethical role models within hospitals.

The principle of responsibility suggests, moreover, that individual trustees should be attentive to the effects the policies and conduct of their hospitals are having on the public's understanding of that hospital and the nature of the health care system. This is the corollary of their duties defined by the principle of accountability.

Writing about journalism and its coverage of the process of democratic governmental representations, Michael Schudson argues that journalists need to act as though they lived in two worlds: the world of the representative system as it might be in some realm of ideal democracy, and the imperfect world of representation as it exists in our actual democracy.[7] He wants the press to champion democracy as it might be, while responding to the realities of democracy as it is.

I suggest that this dual perspective may also apply to hospital trustees. Of course, trustees must live in the real world of our imperfect health care system, and they must cope with the myriad pressures and scarcities hospitals face today. But they should always keep one eye directed toward the far horizon, lest they lose their sense of the whole point of trusteeship and civic service in the first place. The far horizon to which I refer is the promise of an equitable health care system that gives high priority to public health and health promotion, building the social capital of the communities of which the hospital is a part, developing health literacy, and addressing the long-term care needs of chronically ill and disabled people.[8]

Hospital trustees today have an extraordinary opportunity and responsibility that they seem not to recognize. It is the task of creating a governance system for hospitals, and indeed for all health care institutions, that is more inclusive, empowering, and accountable to the interests, needs, and voices of those who are today marginalized and effectively silent. This is the promise of trusteeship as representation in American health care.

NOTES

1. Bruce Jennings and Daniel Callahan, eds., *Representation and Responsibility: Exploring Legislative Ethics* (New York: Plenum Press, 1985).

2. It is questionable how much longer the media or the press can continue to perform this binding function, for economic and commercial forces seem to be fragmenting and polarizing news organizations like never before, and the longstanding ideal of journalistic objectivity is on the wane. For an illuminating general discussion, see Carmen Sirianni and Lewis Friedland, *Civic Innovation in America* (Berkeley: University of California Press, 2001), 186–233.

3. Bruce Jennings, Bradford H. Gray, Virginia A. Sharpe, and Alan R. Fleischman, "Ethics and Trusteeship for Healthcare: Hospital Board Service in Turbulent Times," *Hastings Center Report (Special Supplement)* 32, no. 4 (July–August 2002).

4. Hanna F. Pitkin, *The Concept of Representation* (Berkeley: University of California Press, 1967).

5. Cf. J. Roland Pennock, *Democratic Political Theory* (Princeton, N.J.: Princeton University Press, 1979), 309–62; Robert A. Dahl, *A Preface to Democratic Theory* (Chicago: University of Chicago Press, 1956); and Peter Bachrach, *The Theory of Democratic Elitism* (Boston: Little, Brown, 1967).

6. The ethics of representation is a relatively underdeveloped field. Two important attempts to develop this area are Dennis F. Thompson, *Ethics in Congress: From Individual to Institutional Corruption* (Washington, D.C.: Brookings Institution Press, 1995); and Bruce Jennings and Daniel Callahan, *The Ethics of Legislative Life* (Hastings-on-Hudson, N.Y.: Hastings Center, 1985). See also Amy Gutmann and Dennis F. Thompson, "The Theory of Legislative Ethics," in *Representation and Responsibility*, ed. Jennings and Callahan, 167–95; and Daniel Callahan, William Green, Bruce Jennings, and Martin Linsky, *Congress and the Media: The Ethical Connection* (Hastings-on-Hudson, N.Y.: Hastings Center, 1985).

7. Michael Schudson, *The News Media and the Democratic Process*, Wye Resource Paper (New York: Aspen Institute, 1983).

8. Sirianni and Friedland, *Civic Innovation in America*, 138–85.

9

ETHICAL DIMENSIONS OF TRUSTEESHIP ON THE BOARDS OF CATHOLIC HOSPITALS AND SYSTEMS

Charles J. Dougherty

CATHOLIC HOSPITALS AND SYSTEMS

Catholic health care facilities constitute a sizable portion of American health care. In 1999, there were 569 hospitals, 319 long-term care facilities, 62 health care systems, and 74 other health-related organizations under Catholic sponsorship. (These Catholic entities have 258 sponsors, primarily religious congregations of women and men, but including dioceses and organizations of lay people.) Of all religiously sponsored not-for-profit hospitals, 94 percent are Catholic.[1] Taken together, Catholic health care facilities are the single largest group of not-for-profit health care facilities under a single form of sponsorship.[2] Put another way, Catholic hospitals constitute the largest private-sector effort to deliver health services in the United States.

Compared with all nonfederal U.S. hospitals in 1997, Catholic hospitals accounted for 14 to 16 percent of all the following activities and measures: number of beds (14.6 percent), admissions (15.3 percent), inpatient days (14.9 percent), emergency visits (14.2 percent), total outpatient visits (15.8 percent), inpatient surgeries (16 percent), births recorded (14.7 percent), full-time-equivalent employees (14.8 percent), total payroll (14.9 percent), and total expenses (14.9 percent).[3]

The organizational profile of a Catholic hospital is distinctive. Although there has been a push toward system affiliation throughout the hospital sector, Catholic hospitals are far more likely to be members of systems. Fully 79 percent of Catholic hospitals have a system affiliation, compared with 38 percent of other not-for-profits and 62 percent of investor-owned hospitals.

Of the ten largest hospital corporations in the U.S., five are Catholic: the Daughters of Charity National Health System, Catholic Health Initiatives, Catholic Healthcare West, Catholic Healthcare Network, and Mercy Health Systems.[4] Catholic hospitals tend to be larger than other hospitals, have longer lengths of stay, and are more likely to serve as teaching sites for medical education compared with their peers. They are also distinctive in a more substantive way. A recent study examined the prevalence of compassionate care services at American hospitals. These services were defined as home health, organized social work services, outpatient social work services, emergency social work services, pastoral care, long-term care, hospice, volunteer services, ethics committee, and patient representative services. Compared with both not-for-profit and investor-owned hospitals, Catholic hospitals were found to offer significantly more compassionate care services.[5]

TRUSTEE RESPONSIBILITIES

Given the size and importance of Catholic health care on the American scene, it is useful to examine the special ethical challenges of trusteeship in this context. Catholic hospital trustees share many of the same governance and ethical responsibilities faced by trustees on other not-for-profit hospital and system boards. Like trustees of all corporations, Catholic hospital trustees have a fiduciary responsibility to act in the best interest of the organization they serve. Likewise, they are responsible for selecting, evaluating, and replacing top management and for determining levels of compensation. They provide the same types of financial, legal, and reporting oversight. Trustees regularly review operating statistics, budget performance data, financial statements, and capital planning data.[6] They approve and revise strategic plans. Ultimately, trustees are responsible for policies and practices to ensure the highest and most consistent quality of care for patients.

Most important, along with their peers at other not-for-profit hospital boards, they must struggle with the multiple dimensions of "mission versus margin." Not-for-profits have two bottom lines: performance with respect to the charitable purpose of the organization and financial performance.

In the contemporary health care arena, this dual responsibility involves multiple challenges. First is dealing with increasingly fierce levels of competition between hospitals, both for-profits and not-for-profits. Trustees must strike a delicate balance, learning the new skills of competition without unlearning the traditional skills of compassion. They must do what it takes to thrive in the marketplace without losing the corporation's soul. Trustees must take the lead in developing and sustaining an organizational culture that focuses on charitable intent and community benefit so that the quotidian demands of the marketplace do not erode the organization's founding intent. They must help to identify, develop, and reward leaders who can articulate and act on this dual vision and who can find ways of infusing it practically throughout various units of a complex organization.

Trustees at Catholic hospitals or systems must also identify the various communities served by the hospital or system, measure the health status and needs of those communities, and devise creative ways of addressing unmet needs. At this time in our nation, with its powerful and sophisticated medical armamentarium alongside a vast and growing population of uninsured and underinsured patients, trustees must develop strategies to provide free care without committing institutional suicide.

Finally, trustees at Catholic institutions face the same pressures their not-for-profit hospital peers face in a rapidly consolidating health care delivery system. Proposals for joint ventures, mergers, acquisitions, sales, and closures all must be examined for their strategic wisdom and scrutinized throughout the endless variety of details they embody. Trustees must ensure that any changes in corporate organization that they approve are consistent with the charitable intent of the organization and serve the health care needs of the community.[7]

Hence, the general ethical principles of trusteeship apply to Catholic hospital trustees. They must be faithful to mission, ensure that patients and communities are well served, and act as responsible stewards of the institution's material and human resources. The fact that the institutions they serve also have a specific faith-based mission, however, means that the ethical responsibilities of trustees at Catholic hospitals are enhanced, particularly in the area of fidelity to mission.

RELIGIOUS SPONSORSHIP

In addition to the fiduciary responsibilities that Catholic hospital trustees share with others, they have certain responsibilities that are specific to Catholic health care. The source of these duties is the mission of Catholic hospitals. Broadly speaking, that mission takes its inspiration from the healing ministry of Jesus Christ, the explicit tenets of Catholic medical ethics and social teaching, and the long tradition of spiritually motivated service to sick and poor people by Catholic institutions and individuals.

The healing activities of Jesus Christ are documented in the Christian gospels and are well known. There are textual descriptions of Christ's cures of leprosy, blindness, lameness, deafness, muteness, paralysis, fever, hemorrhage, a withered hand, epilepsy, dropsy, a severed ear, and mental illness (via exorcism). Even the dead are returned to life. These curative acts of Christ—miracles for believers—helped to create an important and enduring association between health care and Christian faith.

The Catholic Church has a highly articulate and long-standing tradition of medical ethics.[8] This tradition shares much with the Hippocratic tradition of Western medicine and with contemporary secular medical ethics. It does, however, embody certain distinctive positions having to do with the meaning of life, and hence of death, and with the significance of the body and sexuality. In addition, Catholic medical ethics has developed and refined distinctive analytic tools such as the distinction between ordinary and extraordinary care, the doctrine of double effect, and the principle of cooperation.

Catholic social teaching during the past century has emphasized justice in public life. This emphasis has given rise to affirmations of the rights of workers (including health care workers), a view that access to health care is a human right, and a preferential option for poor and marginalized people. The preferential option has reinforced the commitment of Catholic health care providers to serve uninsured patients and those with stigmatized illnesses.[9]

Most American Catholic hospitals are sponsored by the religious congregations of women and men who established them, or by their successor organizations. Many of these congregations were started by charismatic individuals whose founding spiritual intent included care for the dying, sick, and abandoned. For example, the founder of the Sisters of Charity was Elizabeth Seton, now recognized by the Catholic Church as the first American-born saint. In the early nineteenth century, she established schools, orphanages, child care centers, and hospitals with a special commitment to poor and sick people. Generations of women from this congregation have sustained this vision, and with it, numerous Catholic hospitals.

Trustees of Catholic hospitals and systems have a general obligation to be aware of these elements of the mission of Catholic health care and to foster them in their decision making. Not all trustees of Catholic hospitals are themselves Catholic. Hence, not all trustees will identify with all these values as individuals. Nevertheless, their fiduciary responsibility as trustees is to advance these faith-based values in the organizations they serve.

There are two dimensions of Catholic health care in which this general obligation of trustees becomes more concrete. First is through the relationship of particular hospitals and hospital systems to their specific religious sponsor. This fidelity to a specific mission also becomes more concrete with respect to hospitals' explicit relationship to the Catholic Church. This is expressed through the authority of Catholic bishops in the dioceses in which Catholic hospitals are located and often through the application of a document developed by American Catholic bishops to articulate the aspirations and rules governing Catholic hospitals: *The Ethical and Religious Directives for Catholic Health Care Services.*[10]

The governance of every hospital involves a delicate balancing of power. There is the legal authority and responsibility of the board. If the hospital is in a system, that authority is limited and shaped by the hospital's obligations to the system. There is considerable power in the medical staff and its organizations, especially through processes of credentialing. Nurses and other professional constituencies that work in hospitals have interests that command attention. There may be unions and union contracts. There is considerable power and influence in other community institutions that a hospital relates to in significant ways—insurers, managed care plans, physicians' groups, and the like. There is the power of public opinion. There are numerous regulatory bodies whose power to affect the daily operations and strategic planning of hospitals is enormous. And there are the blind but inexorable forces of local markets that can be so important in determining options for services offered, populations served, partnerships with other providers, and even hospital survival.

In addition to all of these governance realities, Catholic hospitals have clearly defined relationships to sponsoring organizations that further shape the responsibilities of trustees. Religious sponsorship can take three forms: that of a religious congregation, of a diocese, or of a religiously motivated association of lay people. In the American Catholic experience, the first has been the dominant model. The vast majority of Catholic hospitals were founded by religious congregations of women and men—the Daughters of Charity, the Sisters of Mercy, the Alexian Brothers, for example. These sponsoring organizations have their own particular charisms—charitable traditions and spiritual emphases that have shaped the history and ethos of their congregation and the institutions they have established.

In church law (canon law), each congregation is a religious institute, that is, a voluntary organization of individuals for a religious purpose. Official church recognition makes the institute a public juridic person, declaring that the institute's works are done in the name of the church and conferring a status within the church not unlike that of a civil corporation in secular society. American religious institutes then form not-for-profit corporations to define themselves in civil law. Typically, the not-for-profit organization that is the religious institute is a separate entity from the not-for-profit corporation formed to organize and operate a hospital or a hospital system. Nevertheless, the sponsoring religious organization maintains a special status on the not-for-profit hospital board to ensure that the board continues to carry out the religious mission of the congregation itself.[11]

Thus a religious congregation is a public juridic person to the Church and a nonprofit corporation to the state. Typically this entity is the sponsor of the nonprofit hospital or system corporation.

Although this is not mandated explicitly by canon law, religious institutes have typically ensured their stewardship of hospital corporations by the use of reserve powers. These reserve powers, as the name implies, limit the hospital board's ability to act independently in certain areas and relegates decisions in these areas to the religious congregation. Powers are typically reserved in three areas. First, reserve powers generally prevent the board from changing its fundamental articles of incorporation or its bylaws without the approval of the sponsor. Second, reserve powers generally give the sponsor the right to select board trustees and in some cases key hospital executives. In practice, this power gives the sponsor the right to appoint members of its own religious congregation to the board, as well as to select lay board members—whose numbers have increased dramatically during the past several decades. Finally, reserve powers govern property and its disposition. Much of this last arena is in fact controlled by the church. In canon law, the sale of church property is considered "alienation." Not only do sponsors reserve to themselves the authority to alienate property; they also are obliged to obtain approval for significant alienations (at present, amounts of more than $3 million) from the Vatican itself. Reserve powers also typically control the distribution of hospital assets in the event of merger, sale, or closure.[12]

Although the existence and magnitude of reserve powers may seem a significant diminution of the authority of hospital boards and their trustees, most of these reserve powers are rarely invoked. Aside from the important but episodic function of selecting new board members, in day-to-day practice, the real work of the sponsor occurs through the religious sisters and brothers who are sponsor-designated members of hospital and system boards. In addition to their general responsibility as trustees, their specific role is to inspire, to recall the board to the charitable intentions of the hospital and the religious congregation that founded it, and to encourage the assessment of decisions in terms of the hospital's mission. In other words, though reserve powers give the religious sponsor legal control over the organization in extraordinary circumstances, their ordinary work involves the influence of religious example and aspiration. Looked at from the board perspective, the obligation of the hospital trustee is to receive and accept that influence as part of his or her fiduciary responsibility to the institution. In this manner, the trustees share stewardship of the hospital's religious mission.

CHANGING SPONSORSHIPS

Unfortunately, even with the dedicated service of members of religious congregations who have made this model work on behalf of the patients and communities they have served, congregationally based sponsorship is in its twilight. The religious institutes are facing declining numbers, aging populations, and a consequent shortage of leadership to sustain these sponsorship obligations. Because of this and because of a greater understanding in the church of the role of the laity, there has been a significant increase in leadership roles for lay people. In 1998, about 70 percent of Catholic health care systems and 91 percent of Catholic health care facilities were headed by laypeople.[13] This change is captured by the experience of Mercy Sister Mary Agnes Connor, who first joined a Catholic hospital board in 1959 and offered the following reflection in 1994:

> When I first became a trustee, the only members of the corporation board were the major superior and her counsel. An advisory board of laypersons contributed their expertise in medicine, law, banking, construction, and other areas.
>
> Today the laity are full members of the board just as the sisters are. Laypeople participate on all the board committees. They also feel more responsible for the mission and values of the organization than in the early days when those concerns were considered the responsibility of the sisters.[14]

Even this model of the sisters sharing authority with lay people cannot long continue in light of their declining numbers. Edward J. Connors, past president of Mercy Health Systems, has written, "Sadly, all reasonable signs point to the inability of most—if not all—Catholic religious congregations to continue as sponsor-owners much beyond another decade if indeed that long."[15] The goal of congregational sponsors and their trustee partners now is to continue to inculcate the values of the founding religious institute throughout the hospital so that they endure even as new methods of sponsorship evolve. There are many efforts under way to accomplish this goal, for example, efforts to professionalize the role of mission leader in Catholic hospitals.[16]

Alternative models of sponsorship can take two general forms. First, a Catholic hospital might be operated as a diocesan entity with a board appointed by and responsible to the local bishop. Some American Catholic hospitals are organized like this, and their numbers may grow. More likely, however, is growth in a second model in which lay individuals, having formed an association with a religious purpose, are recognized by the Catholic Church as a public juridic person. The hospital board itself or some subset of the board becomes the sponsor. In these arrangements, the sponsors could be all or mostly all laypeople.[17]

A recent example of a move in this direction occurred in the creation of Catholic Health Initiatives (CHI) in 1996. Three large Catholic systems (the Sisters of Charity Health Care Systems, Franciscan Health System, and Catholic Health Corporation) merged to become CHI, one of the five largest Catholic systems in the nation. Before the merger, each system had its own sponsor; the Sisters of Charity and the Franciscan Sisters in the first two cases and in the case of the Catholic Health Corporation a public juridic person that was not linked to a single congregation. CHI chose to adopt Catholic Health Corporation's sponsorship for the new organization, and it formed a public juridic person that is a board composed half of laypeople and half of vowed religious from a number of different congregations.

It is likely there will be additional experimentation with this model of sponsorship. Such experimentation will have an impact on the role and responsibilities of trustees of Catholic hospitals. But if the aspirations of current sponsors and trustees are realized, changes in sponsorship will not affect the fundamental mission of Catholic health care facilities.

BISHOPS AND THE *DIRECTIVES*

Whether the sponsoring association is religious, lay, or some combination, the ministry of all Catholic health facilities and services within a local diocese is subject to the oversight and authority of the diocesan bishop.[18] This is evidenced in the bishop's authority to control the designation of "Catholic." Each local diocesan bishop decides which organizations may bear this designation.[19] He can recognize new entities as Catholic. He can also remove this designation when, in his assessment, an organization has changed its mission or behavior and is no longer serving the general mission of the church.

When working with Catholic hospitals, bishops will typically refer to *The Ethical and Religious Directives for Catholic Health Care Services*, published by the National Conference of Catholic Bishops in 1966 and revised in 1994. The purpose of the *Directives* is to assert the church's teaching on the dignity of human persons in the health care context and to provide "authoritative guidance on certain moral issues that face Catholic health care today."[20] The *Directives* contains sections on the social responsibility of Catholic health care services, the pastoral and spiritual responsibility of Catholic health care, the professional–patient relationship, issues in caring for those at the beginning of life, issues in caring for the dying, and issues in forming new partnerships with other health care organization. It includes an appendix on principles governing the limits of cooperation with activities the church holds are wrong. The last section on partnerships and the appendix on cooperation are new in the 1994 edition and express concerns and offer guidance about the new world of joint ventures, mergers, and acquisitions.

Each section of the *Directives* begins with general principles and aspirations and then sets out directives that offer specific moral guidance. Individual directives include material on the relatively settled matters (for Catholics) of providing sacraments to the sick and the dying, affirming a patient's free and informed consent to treatment, and forbidding abortion. Issues that are more controverted within Catholic medical ethics circles are also addressed, such as the treatment of ectopic pregnancies, the range of care for victims of rape, and the withdrawal of hydration and nutrition from the irreversibly comatose.[21] The *Directives* is regarded as definitive teaching in Catholic health care and is used in both clinical decision making and policy setting. Catholic bishops are certain to refer to the *Directives* when approached with ethical problems in these areas. In spite of the relative specificity of many of the directives, the expanding power of medicine, the variety of clinical and social circumstances, and the need for prudence in applying rules to cases dictate the need for moral judgment. Even the most explicit directives must be interpreted and applied through hospital policies and practices.

There are at least three implications here for trustees on Catholic hospital boards. First and most obvious, they should be familiar with the *Directives* and their applications. This is more challenging than it sounds, because many lay board members do not have the intellectual grounding in Catholic medical ethics that the *Directives* presupposes. This implies an obligation for continuing education. Second, trustees should develop and maintain a relationship of openness and trust with the local bishop—and for trustees on system boards, with all the bishops in the dioceses in which their hospitals are located. Again, this is more challenging than it may seem. Many bishops are not as knowledgeable about medicine, health policy, and the economics of contemporary hospital care as could be desired. Third, board members considering controversial clinical or corporate decisions, especially decisions that may have an impact on the Catholic identity of their organization, should consult early and often in the process with the bishop or his representative.[22]

PROHIBITED SERVICES

There are three sensitive areas in which trustees have the responsibility to be especially attentive to the *Directives* and to the local bishop. The first area includes what are referred to as prohibited services. These include abortion, sterilization, contraception, in vitro fertilization, and assisted suicide. Second is the controversial question of the relationship between Catholic hospitals and for-profit entities. Can a Catholic hospital or its subsidiaries be operated for profit? The third area has to do with partnering: joint ventures, mergers, and acquisitions. What kind of corporate combinations are consistent with maintaining a Catholic identity?

Directive 45 states: "Abortion (that is, the directly intended termination of pregnancy before viability or the directly intended destruction of a viable fetus) is never permitted."[23] This is probably the most definitive moral prohibition in the Directives. Closely related in temper is Directive 60: "Catholic health care institutions may never condone or participate in euthanasia or assisted suicide in any way."[24] These two prohibitions are based on the Catholic view that human life in all its stages has a divinely conferred dignity. Neither the unborn nor the dying may be killed directly. The banning of sterilization, contraception, and in vitro fertilization follows from church teaching on sexuality (except in the last case, if fertilized eggs or embryos are destroyed; then the basis again is respect for life). Although the teaching in the Directives is definitive in these areas as well, there is a larger measure of toleration in practice for association with other health care entities that offer or fund these services.

A recent controversy that may prove ethically challenging for some trustees of Catholic hospitals involves the acquisition of non-Catholic hospitals. When this occurs, the Directives become effective in the new entity, for it has either become Catholic itself or is operated by a Catholic entity. Prohibited services that may have been offered by the other hospital before the acquisition will no longer be available. In some cases, before the completion of the acquisition, the non-Catholic entity establishes or facilitates establishment of another corporation or entity through which some of these services may continue to be provided outside Catholic auspices. Typically this involves contraception and sterilization and is referred to in Catholic circles as a "carve out." The prohibited services are removed, carved out, from the acquisition so that the resulting Catholic entity has no supervisory or financial relationship to them. This protects the ethical integrity of the Catholic entity and yet allows for access to what many (perhaps most) believe are morally permissible services.[25]

Because of the perceived difference in the gravity of the moral issue, Catholic entities do not cooperate similarly with abortion services. (Nor will they likely do so with assisted suicide, should it become widely available.) Thus circumstances can arise in which hospital acquisition by a Catholic hospital or system will restrict access to abortion. Some groups have expressed concerns about this, especially when it involves Catholic acquisition of a sole provider in a community. In these cases, abortion was available in the community before the acquisition; it is not available afterward. The magnitude of this problem is debatable. Abortion rights advocates claim it as a serious problem; the Catholic Health Association has produced data showing that it seldom happens.[26]

Of course, those who do not accept the Catholic view of these matters, especially advocates of abortion rights, present their own position as a moral argument turning on the claim of a right to choose abortion. Moreover, some see the loss of access to prohibited services as a disservice to the health care needs of a community. Trustees on a Catholic hospital board may personally share this view of abortion rights or may have some sympathy for the concern about restricted access to legal services. This might create a crisis of conscience for an individual board member. But continued service on a Catholic hospital board requires fidelity to the institution's mission. Board members are bound to support the application of the *Directives* in these matters. If abortion is the grave moral wrong that Catholic teaching holds it to be, there can be no right of access to it for an individual or a community. It is not a morally legitimate health care service. According to the *Directives*, "Catholic health care does not offend the rights of individual conscience by refusing to provide or permit medical procedures that are judged morally wrong by the teaching authority of the Church."[27]

Aside from one's views of abortion and Catholicism, no religious organization should be expected to compromise on such deeply held religious and ethical beliefs. The prudence of any hospital acquisition can be debated, and should be, by any number of voices, including those of the communities affected. But if a hospital is acquired by a Catholic health care provider, the *Directives* will apply. The trustees of the Catholic board are bound to apply them.

THE FOR-PROFIT ISSUE

Catholic doctrine does not prohibit Catholic hospitals from partnering with for-profit hospitals or for-profit hospital chains.[28] Canon law does not even mandate that an activity be not-for-profit in order to be sponsored by the church. The important issue from the church's point of view is where the profits go. If they are applied to another recognized charitable purpose, there is no canonical problem in a for-profit undertaking.[29] This is the justification for the use of for-profit subsidiaries by Catholic hospitals and hospital boards; namely, that the profits from these subsidiaries go to sustain the charitable purpose of the not-for-profit parent organization. This distinction is similar to that in American corporate law between for-profit and not-for-profit organizations. The distinction does not have to do with the generation of profits themselves but rather with the mode of their distribution. Peter Campbell makes the point this way:

> "Not-for-profit" corporations, which came into being for ecclesiastical or charitable purposes have always been allowed to make a "profit," although law prohibits individuals from profiting. The distinction between for-profit and not-for-

profit corporations is not an ability to make money, but rather what they each can do with their net earnings. Without "profits," not-for-profit corporations obviously could not long continue.[30]

The nub of the argument about the relationship of Catholic health care to for-profit health care has not turned, therefore, on the semantics of whether an operating margin is really a profit, nor on any particulars of canon law. It has turned instead on an assessment of the organizational culture that is created when health care organizations are operated for profit, particularly by modern publicly traded, investor-owned, multi-hospital corporations. In these contexts, stockholders have legal rights to private inurement, and the corporation is obliged to provide them. The corporation is under the quarterly performance pressure of stock markets. These facts of life for investor-owned for-profits create a particular organizational culture. This culture is not wrong in itself. Much of the American economy operates this way. Churches, charities, and other non-for-profits depend on the wealth this economy generates.

The vexing question has been: Can an entity be both for-profit in this sense and Catholic at the same time?[31] The general answer that has emerged within Catholic health care and the official position of the Catholic Health Association is negative. An organization cannot be both a publicly traded, investor-owned for-profit corporation and also be Catholic.[32] The dominant view is that the organizational culture of such a for-profit entity inevitably will overwhelm its charitable purpose as Catholic. Trustees on an investor-owned for-profit corporation board have a fiduciary responsibility to maximize benefits to stockholders. Thus, reorganization or "conversion" to this for-profit status would put Catholic hospital trustees and top executives in an impossible bind: being obliged at once to pursue a charitable and spiritual purpose and at the same time maximize profits for passive investors.[33]

PARTNERS AND COOPERATION

The for-profit issue is just one instance of larger questions about partnering. Changes in health care delivery and financing have forced hospital closures, consolidations, and partnering (joint ventures, mergers, and acquisitions) throughout the hospital sector. Catholic hospitals are not exceptions. In the first half of the 1990s, for example, forty-two Catholic hospitals were sold or merged and are no longer Catholic. Seven merged and retained their Catholic identity. Twelve Catholic hospitals closed their doors altogether.[34]

Multiple difficulties are associated with any partnering relationship between two organizations. Organizations have cultures. Their trustees and executives have personalities. Cultures and personalities at two different hospitals may or may not coexist easily. Joint ventures between Catholic hospitals share all these challenges, as well as those associated with relationships between differing sponsors. In Catholic-to-Catholic partnerships, there is a shared foundation of church teaching and the application of the *Directives*. Nevertheless, histories of competition and mutual suspicion, a sense of loss of identity, or a feeling of being trapped into partnerships by unfavorable market realities can make even these relationships risky ventures.[35]

Because of geographic patterns and the idiosyncrasies of local markets, Catholic hospitals cannot partner only with one another. The chief executive officer of a Catholic hospital in the Midwest remarked, "If we just do business with Catholics, we're not going to be around."[36] Thus, in addition to the general challenges of hospital partnering and the additional difficulties of blending sponsorships in Catholic-to-Catholic ventures, trustees on Catholic hospital boards are often faced with the demands of partnering with hospitals that have other religious traditions, or (in most cases) none at all. There is considerable unease in Catholic circles about the long-term implications of such relationships, particularly when the merger is fifty-fifty or when the Catholic partner has a minority position. These "arranged marriages" may be the solution to maintaining Catholic identity in a highly competitive and consolidating marketplace. However, they may be the first step in the loss of an organization's Catholic identity.[37] As in so many decisions of this sort, the outcome (and the devil) may lie in the details of the arrangements.

Whatever the details, trustees on Catholic hospital boards have to bear in mind *Directive 69* when contemplating such partnerships: "When a Catholic health care institution is participating in a partnership that may be involved in activities judged morally wrong by the Church, the Catholic institution should limit its involvement in accord with the moral principles governing cooperation."[38] This reference to the principle of cooperation anticipates the appendix that was added to the *Directives* on this topic.[39] The principle of cooperation is an analytic tool to help define the kinds and limits of permissible cooperation with another party who is engaged in wrongdoing.[40] It is frequently used to determine the acceptability of partnerships with other hospitals who have some policies or practices that are incompatible with Catholic teaching. *Directive 45* states that this analysis may not be used to justify the provision of abortion services by Catholic health care institutions, demonstrating again the moral gravity the church attaches to the destruction of fetal life.[41]

The principle of cooperation is appealed to frequently, however, in crafting partnerships between Catholic hospitals and other entities that provide tubal ligation, contraception, or in vitro fertilization or that may themselves have a relationship with abortion (perhaps through a managed care or insurance plan). A Catholic hospital, for example, may find it desirable to develop a joint venture, say, a home health care organization, with a nondenominational community hospital. If that hospital offers in vitro fertilization services and has a managed care contract that links it to an abortion clinic, trustees on the Catholic hospital may be concerned about the permissibility of their cooperation with the community hospital. The principle of cooperation offers a framework through which these ethical issues can be examined in an organized fashion. It is also a common platform for the initiation of discussions with the local bishop.

The first fundamental distinction required for application of the principle of cooperation is that between formal and material cooperation. In an act of formal cooperation, the agent cooperating intends, that is, deliberately wills, to perform the same action as the wrongdoer (technically, intends the same object as the wrongdoer's activity). Because this amounts to a willful choice of evil, formal cooperation is never permitted. Hence, this framework for analysis is sometimes referred to as the principle of material cooperation because only material cooperation is permissible, and only certain forms of it. Thus, the first requirement of acceptable cooperation is that the cooperator—the Catholic hospital, in this case—does not want to be involved in an activity that the church considers wrongful but is brought into association with it because it is being conducted or condoned by the partner community hospital. The benefits of partnership may not be used to justify deliberate wrongdoing. Catholicism does not countenance reasoning based on the "lesser of two evils" or the concept that the "ends justify the means." If it is wrong, an act may not be intended either as an end or as a means to an end.

Therefore, in the case at hand, the Catholic hospital board cannot *want* to be associated with the community hospital's in vitro program or its link to abortion. Even the potential benefits of the home health care effort cannot induce the Catholic partner to intend these activities.

The next pertinent distinction involves that between immediate and mediate material cooperation. The former is unacceptable; the latter can be acceptable. In immediate material cooperation, the cooperator—despite his desire not to—performs the very same act as the wrongdoer (technically, the object of the act is the same). For example, if the Catholic hospital in this case does not want to engage in in vitro fertilization but is asked to do so as a condition for the proposed partnership, it could not agree. Despite its refusal of formal cooperation, agreement to do so would constitute immediate material cooperation. This kind of "don't want to but have to" cooperation is not permitted. In rare cases, an exception for duress is recognized.

There has been considerable discussion about what constitutes duress and how extreme the duress may have to be before immediate material cooperation can be justified. The consensus seems to be that justifications by way of duress are rare and must be extreme, perhaps involving the potential for loss of Catholic presence. For example, duress might be raised as a possible justification if the Catholic hospital's inability to partner with the community hospital meant that it would have to close and leave the community without a Catholic provider. Even then, it likely would not provide sufficient justification for providing in vitro fertilizations, given the following additional conditions that determine acceptable material cooperation

If the material cooperation is mediate so that the Catholic partner neither intends nor is directly engaged in the wrongdoing, the cooperation of the Catholic partner may be ethically justified, given two other considerations: proximity and proportionality. First, the Catholic partner must distance itself as far as possible from the wrongdoing. Obviously, this is a matter of degree; the further the distance, the more readily justified the cooperation. This can be accomplished through "carve outs," as indicated above. These arrangements keep the Catholic partner at moral arm's length by removing financial and supervisory control over activities deemed to be wrong.

The second consideration is a proportionality test. The reasons for the partnership, for example, providing needed home health care to the community, must be proportionately grave to justify the degree of cooperation and the gravity of the wrongdoing involved. This is a balancing test, not unlike utilitarian reasoning. But unlike classical utilitarianism, right and wrong are held to exist independent of the test. What is wrong cannot be intended regardless of the balancing of good and evil. The balancing here is to assess the acceptability of cooperation with another agent whose activities are wrongful.

It is clear that these last two considerations involve a great deal of prudential decision making. How close is too close? How much good must be achieved or evil avoided to justify a given level of participation with a given degree of wrongfulness? People of goodwill, including bishops, can and do differ on their assessments of permissible cooperation in particular cases.

In the community hospital case, there would likely be no direct Catholic link to its in vitro program. Hence, there is probably sufficient supervisory and financial distance. The contract with the abortion provider is more problematic. The insurance or managed care plan covering the home health care services could not be the same plan that links the community hospital to the abortion provider, because this financial link would probably be viewed as too close for the Catholic hospital. The development of separate coverage for the home health care services or carving out the link between the Catholic hospital and the abortion provider would be necessary to address the proximity standard.

Application of the proportionality test, as in most cases, is difficult here. Reasonable people may "weigh" the same factors and reach different conclusions. Factors that might shape a determination would include, on the one hand, the degree of need for the home health services, the population to benefit, and the lack of any good alternative for delivery of these services. On the other hand would be the nature of the in vitro services (e.g., are embryos routinely destroyed?), the character of the relationship between the community hospital and the abortion provider, and whether the joint venture would in any way increase or foster existing wrongdoing. Given the right assessments here, the proportionality test might be met.

There is one final aspect of the principle that underscores the discretion that must be used in its application, as well as the need for early involvement of the bishop. Mediate material cooperation that passes the proximity and proportionality tests must also avoid the possibility of scandal, which in this context is not simply a matter of bad public relations. Rather, scandal here means the potential for undermining the faith of believers, eroding the credibility of faith-based institutions, or compromising the church's prophetic responsibility (the duty to speak out against wrongdoing). Bishops and trustees may convince themselves that cooperation in a certain case is morally acceptable and still decide against the partnership because of the potential for the negative effects of scandal.

In this case, for example, all the other tests may have been passed and cooperation with the community hospital may still be judged unacceptable. Suppose, for example, that the in vitro program or the abortion clinic has a very high profile in a small community. Suppose further that one or both have been criticized frequently or been the object of protests by Catholic groups. Suppose the in vitro fertilization service uses multiple fertilization and selective abortion techniques, or the abortion clinic performs late-term abortions. Or, suppose that the Catholic credentials of the hospital are under challenge in the community because of previous controversial decisions or affiliations. In these circumstances, the technical Catholic ethical analysis of right and wrong may change little, but the stakes for alienating believers are immeasurably higher. Then the potential for scandal makes morally unacceptable what would otherwise be morally acceptable cooperation.

It is important to add that this analysis of cooperation is not only applicable to partnerships involving prohibited services. A Catholic hospital may find itself deliberating a potential partnership with another hospital or health care entity that refuses or avoids service to poor and uninsured people, does not accept Medicaid, has substandard working conditions, provides poor pay and benefits to employees, actively advocates against universal access to care, or has a fiercely competitive, commodity-based interpretation of health care. All these positions are incompatible with Catholic teaching. Yet they are widespread in the American health care system, perhaps more widespread than prohibited services. Catholic health care is a part of this world, literally and figuratively. Moral absolutists and other purists sometimes find hypocrisy in the fine reasoning and subtle moral distinctions of the principle of cooperation. However, the principle allows a way for Catholic institutions to maintain their mission and their organizational integrity and yet live and work in a world of diverse moral and nonmoral views. And, it is hoped, make the world better by doing so.

Because of rapid changes in the delivery and financing of health care and the consequent dislocations occurring in the hospital sector, these are trying times for hospital trustees, particularly for those at not-for-profit institutions. It is difficult for conscientious trustees to identify and act on their ethical responsibilities as fiduciary agents for their institutions. Trusteeship on a Catholic hospital or system board introduces additional complications. In some respects, these complications are morally clarifying. The heritage and active involvement of religious sponsors, the authority of bishops, the developed ethical and social teachings, and the specificity of the *Ethical and Religious Directives for Catholic Health Care Services* provide moral guideposts that are unavailable to trustees on other hospital and system boards. However, these same factors can make the ethical responsibility of trustees on Catholic boards and systems even more demanding.

These moral guideposts create more personal and institutional relationships to manage, some of which are rather delicate. Some health services that are legal are morally prohibited for Catholic providers and many issues that are viewed by others as unproblematic are identified as ethical problems. Most important, there is the general challenge of faithfulness to a particular and evolving mission that marks Catholic health care as a significant but nonetheless minority presence in the American health care system.

The Catholic identity of these hospitals and systems will be shaped in the future by changes in sponsorship and by the ways in which church teachings are applied to corporate decision making, particularly in the area of partnering. The fiduciary responsibility to preserve and foster this identity and the mission it expresses is the essential additional ethical responsibility of trustees on boards of Catholic hospitals and systems.

NOTES

1. Kenneth White and James Begun, "How Does Catholic Hospital Sponsorship Affect Services Provided," *Inquiry* 35 (winter 1998–99): 398.
2. Data from the Catholic Health Association, available at www.chausa.org.ABOUTCHA /CHAFACTS.asp.
3. Data from the Catholic Health Association.
4. Melanie Conklin, "Blocking Women's Health Care," *Progressive* 62, no. 1 (1998): 1.
5. White and Begun, "How Does Catholic Hospital Sponsorship Affect Services," 404.
6. American Hospital Association, "Trustees in Transition," *Trustee* 51, no. 7 (1998): 16.
7. Diana Bianco, "Considering Conversion?" *Trustee*, 51, no. 10 (1998): 16–21.
8. Kevin D. O'Rourke and Philip Boyle, *Medical Ethics: Sources of Catholic Teaching* (Saint Louis: Catholic Health Association, 1989).

9. United States Catholic Conference, *Health and Health Care: A Pastoral Letter of the American Catholic Bishops* (Washington, D.C.: United States Catholic Conference, 1981).

10. National Conference of Catholic Bishops, *Ethical and Religious Directives for Catholic Health Care Services* (Washington, D.C.: United States Catholic Conference, 1995).

11. Peter Campbell, "Evolving Sponsorship and Corporate Structures," *Health Progress* 76, no. 6 (1995): 36.

12. Campbell, "Evolving Sponsorship," 40.

13. Michael Place, "Telling Your Story: The Importance of Communications," *Health Progress* 80, no. 3 (1999): 8.

14. Michael Scavotto, "The New Trustee," *Health Progress* 75, no. 4 (1994): 49.

15. Richard McCormick, "The End of Catholic Hospitals?" *America* 179, no. 1 (1998): 5.

16. Mary Kathryn Grant, "Mission at the Millennium," *Health Progress* 80, no. 2 (1999): 18–20.

17. Campbell, "Evolving Sponsorship," 41.

18. Joseph Bernardin, "What Makes a Hospital Catholic: A Response," *America* 174, no. 45 (1999): 11.

19. Francis Morrissey, "Church Law's Role in Collaborations," *Health Progress* 74, no. 9 (1993): 25.

20. National Conference of Catholic Bishops, *Ethical and Religious Directives*, 1.

21. Kevin O'Rourke, "Applying the Directives," *Health Progress* 79, no. 4 (1998): 64–69.

22. Morrisey, "Church Law's Role," 29.

23. National Conference of Catholic Bishops, *Ethical and Religious Directives*, 19.

24. National Conference of Catholic Bishops, *Ethical and Religious Directives*, 23.

25. Deanna Bellandi, "What Hospitals Won't Do for a Merger," *Modern Health Care* 28, no. 39 (1998): 29.

26. Place, "Telling Your Story," 10. See also Conklin, "Blocking Women's Health Care"; Deanna Bellandi, "CHA Counterattacks Study on Mergers," *Modern Health Care* 29, no. 19 (1999): 14–15; as well as Carol Weisman, Amal Khoury, Christopher Cassirer, Virginia A. Sharpe, and Laura Morlock, "The Implications of Affiliations between Catholic and Non-Catholic Health Care Organizations for Availability of Reproductive Services," *Women's Health Issues* 9, no. 3 (1999): 121–34.

27. National Conference of Catholic Bishops, *Ethical and Religious Directives*, 7.

28. Bruce Japsen, "Speakers Defend Catholic, For-Profit Ties," *Modern Health Care* 26, no. 14 (1996): 19.

29. Morrissey, "Church Law's Role," 28.

30. Campbell, "Evolving Sponsorship," 37.

31. James Clifton and Jean de Blois, "Can For-Profit Hospitals Be Catholic," *National Catholic Reporter* 34, no. 6 (1997): 20.

32. Cathy Tokarski, "For Whom the Church Bell Tolls," *Hospitals and Health Networks* 69, no. 20 (1995): 41.

33. Bernardin, "What Makes a Hospital Catholic: A Response," 9.

34. White and Begun, "How Does Catholic Hospital Sponsorship Affect Services," 398.

35. Patricia Sieman, "Joint Sponsorship Requires Risks," *Health Progress* 77, no. 4 (1996): 34.

36. Bruce Japsen, "Church Puts Faith in System Mergers," *Modern Healthcare* 24, no. 23 (1994): 33.

37. McCormick, *End of Catholic Hospitals?* 5–11.

38. National Conference of Catholic Bishops, *Ethical and Religious Directives*, 27.

39. National Conference of Catholic Bishops, *Ethical and Religious Directives*, 29.

40. James Keenan and Thomas Kopfensteiner, "The Principle of Cooperation," *Health Progress* 76, no. 3 (1995): 23–27.

41. National Conference of Catholic Bishops, *Ethical and Religious Directives*, 19.

PART III

Trusteeship in Practice: Decisions and Systems

10

HOSPITAL PARTNERING, SALES, AND FOR-PROFIT CONVERSIONS

Trustees' Responsibility and Perceptions in a Time of Change

Linda Weiss and Bradford H. Gray

Every health care institution has had to take a trip, and it's been very fast and very scary.

—Hospital trustee, discussing a decision

R ecent years have seen unprecedented changes in the ownership and control of nonprofit hospitals. These changes have occurred as health care markets have faced some combination of increased competition, growing pressure from payers (both government and managed care), shifts to outpatient care, and excess capacity. Hospitals' bottom lines have been severely threatened, and many independent hospitals have, as a result, sought the means to become part of larger health care systems—through purchases, mergers, or affiliations—or to sell their assets, possibly to a for-profit firm. In 1997 alone, 627 hospitals were involved in mergers and acquisitions.[1] Between 1994 and 1996, 155 nonprofit hospitals and hospital systems became—through sale or conversion—for-profit, representing a significant increase from prior years.[2] Although the trend has slowed more recently, it has not ended.[3]

Hospital trustees are key players in the sometimes gut-wrenching decisions that lead to these transitions—gut-wrenching because they relate to institutional ownership, autonomy, and survival; and have significant symbolic and practical implications, yet no clear answers. Until recent times, trustees facing difficult decisions could assess alternatives in terms of the best interests of the hospital as an easily defined and identified entity, and they could generally assume that those interests correspond with the best interests of the community. But as the communities that spawned the hospitals relocate, as health care moves outside the hospital walls, and as financial pressures make economic efficiency a necessity, the interests of a hospital—interests such as survival, autonomy, and possibly growth—may not coincide with the interests of other key parties, including those the hospital was originally established to serve. Trustees must sometimes determine anew where priorities lie for the institutions that they hold in trust. Do they continue to reside within the institution, with the bricks and mortar, the name, the patients and staff? Or should trustees now assume a broader health mission—in the words of one trustee we interviewed, "to preserve the community's entitlement to quality health care"— even at the expense of institutional survival?

Methods and Sampling

This chapter is based on open-ended interviews with ninety-eight trustees and chief executive officers (CEOs) at twenty-two hospitals, as described in more detail in chapter 7. Two sets of hospitals were included. The bulk of these interviews were at sixteen New York–area hospitals selected at random from a sample stratified into four groups: academic medical centers (n = 4), major teaching hospitals (n = 6), urban community hospitals (n = 1),[4] and suburban community hospitals (n = 5). Of these sixteen hospitals, five had a religious affiliation and nine were in urban centers.

Our New York–area interviews covered a number of topics, including views of trustee responsibility and hospital mission. There was no planned focus on ownership, control, and partnering issues, but because of the frequency with which hospitals faced these issues and their importance to affected institutions, these topics became a very significant part of many of the interviews we conducted with the nonprofit trustees and CEOs.

Interviews in the second sample, the "conversion sample," which includes six hospitals in the eastern United States that recently considered sale or conversion to for-profit status, were focused primarily on this particular decision and the control and ownership issues surrounding it. Hospitals were identified for the conversion sample through the trade press, supplemented by expert advice. Selection was based on a number of criteria, including the different solutions they chose (two chose to remain nonprofit, four did not). We also looked for diversity in location and type of institutions, options considered, the processes used to reach a decision, and the controversy surrounding it. Of the six, two had religious affiliations, two were teaching hospitals, two were community hospitals, and two were specialty hospitals. One hospital was owned by a university.[5] Four hospitals in the conversion sample were in urban centers; two were suburban.

At both sets of hospitals, we sought to interview the CEO, board chair, and three other trustees selected by the chair and/or CEO—one each with particular interest or expertise regarding: (1) financial matters, (2) patient care concerns, and (3) the community. These criteria were used to ensure that we would be exposed to a range of perspectives and viewpoints. Virtually all of the interviews were face-to-face. Notes were taken during the interviews; most were also tape recorded (with permission) to ensure accuracy and allow for the use of quotations.

In the following sections, we cover what we learned regarding why and how the partnering/sale/conversion issue arose, what factors the boards had considered, what kind of arrangements were made, and how participants view their decisions in retrospect. We generally use the terms "partnering" or "affiliation" to refer to all these kinds of arrangements. Throughout the discussion, we have tried to emphasize *trustees'* perceptions of their options and choices and the values they bring to their decisions.

FREQUENCY OF AFFILIATION ACTIVITY

During the past several years, the development of partnering and affiliation arrangements has been a prominent concern among New York City–area hospitals. Through mergers, sales, and other types of affiliation arrangements, most area hospitals have become part of some sort of local system, which range in size from two to thirty or more hospitals. This affiliation activity is evident in the data we collected; 59 percent of the trustees and CEOs interviewed in 1998–99 as part of the New York sample, representing thirteen of the sixteen hospitals included, indicated that partnering or affiliation issues were one of the two most important issues that their hospital had faced in the last year alone. At some of these hospitals, trustees had been deliberating about which partner and type of partnership agreement to enter into. At others, trustees had moved on to issues related to the implementation of agreements, including integrating services and seeking efficiencies. Of the three hospitals where partnering was not mentioned as an important issue in the previous year, two had joined with systems several years back, and the other one was just beginning a search for partners. That hospital had not felt pressure before because, being in a small city some distance from the closest hospital, it was "the only game in town." Of those that had already considered partnering, only one had decided *not* to do so. According to the CEO there, trustees felt the institution was sufficiently large already and that further bargaining power or economies of scale were not likely to occur.

Hospitals in the conversion sample were also located in areas with significant affiliation activity. Trustees at each of these hospitals mentioned that their own hospital's need for change was in part a response to that activity. According to one trustee whose hospital sold to a for-profit company:

> The affiliation of [three other hospitals] set the tone for the rest of the town. . . . The board [here] said OK, this is formidable competition. They're going to have negotiating strength with HMOs [health maintenance organizations]. We've got one hospital; we're in one location. They [the merged institutions] were taking the metropolitan area into consideration. When you looked at their different locations, you saw a different competitor. You saw a much different competitor. [Trustee from an urban teaching hospital]

At another institution in the conversion sample, the former CEO commented that "once the merger of [Hospitals A, B, and C] occurred, everyone started talking to everyone else."

TRUSTEE INVOLVEMENT IN PARTNERING DECISIONS

Although hospital CEOs and other executive staff play significant roles in partnering, the ultimate decision is the responsibility of the trustees. In the New York sample, the majority of trustees who faced partnering decisions considered them to have been among the most important faced by the board. At hospitals in the conversion sample as well, everyone we interviewed considered the decision regarding sale or conversion to for-profit to have been the most important issue (basically the only issue) the board faced during the year preceding the decision. Several trustees at both sets of institutions commented that the partnering/sale issue was the most important decision the hospital had *ever* faced.

As was mentioned above, board members took key roles in the development of partnering arrangements. At five of the six hospitals in our conversion sample, at least one of the trustees interviewed spent ten or more hours a week on board-related work in the year preceding the decision. At four of the six hospitals, at least one trustee spent twenty hours or more a week, with two trustees taking on board responsibility essentially or actually as a full-time job. (in one case, the board chair became acting CEO for six months and worked days, evenings, and weekends). The chair of one hospital that sold to a for-profit lamented: "I must have spent thirty hours a week. I didn't go anywhere without a phone or fax. I never spent more time on anything in my life. . . . It drove me nuts" [chair of an urban teaching hospital].

With this kind of time commitment, it is not surprising that, at a number of institutions, board members were instrumental in the development of partnering strategies, including setting minimum criteria, making initial contacts and then negotiating with potential partners, or initiating consideration of a request for proposals (RFP) process.

It is, likewise, not surprising that the decisions were highly emotional, affecting some of the trustees—particularly those considering sale to a for-profit company—deeply. According to one trustee whose board decided to sell to a for-profit: "I struggled with this until the day before the final vote. I [agreed] with it all along because I was seeing what we had to do. But I hurt the entire trip, and I struggled the entire trip" [trustee, urban teaching hospital].

Reasons for Partnering

We were told in our interviews that agreements with other institutions, agreements that included governance, autonomy, and financial responsibility—in some cases ownership—had been sought for a diverse set of reasons, most of which had an economic basis. These reasons include declining revenues, limited access to needed capital, pressures arising from the affiliations or mergers of competing institutions, an inability to cope with the changes that have occurred in health care, the hope of expanding the patient base or attracting the highest-quality physicians, and/or the belief that these different arrangements would improve efficiencies in scale and scope and thus improve their financial strength. A large academic medical center in our sample was facing deficits predicted to be greater than $50 million in each of the coming years. Without a merger, one trustee told us, "draconian expense cuts" would have been necessary. According to trustees at other sample institutions:

Independence is revered here. This trait is seen in the minds of many people, including trustees . . . [but] one can't just consider what's going on in this hospital, you have to consider the environment it's operating in. If all other hospitals have aggregated into larger systems, you can be out of business because all the contracts will have gone to them. [CEO, suburban community hospital]

The realities of the environment we're operating in argued so persuasively that this [merger] really had to happen. You say, "Well, why?" You can't save that much money in the laundry or purchasing or prescription drugs. But ultimately—we'll have to go very slowly—but ultimately the efficiencies will argue very persuasively that this was the right thing to do. [Chair, academic medical center]

To affect efficiencies, to become a more important health care provider, to be able to negotiate with managed care providers with greater strength, to build on each other's strength, to in some cases regionalize . . . by bringing [the hospitals] together to create something stronger and more able to serve our community and more attractive to centers of excellence. [Chair, urban teaching hospital]

Managed care was a concern of trustees at a number of hospitals. Some highlighted what they saw as a divide-and-conquer strategy of HMOs, which negotiated low reimbursement rates with one hospital and then required other hospitals to match that rate or lose their contracts. A number of respondents felt the only way to counter the power of HMOs was to join together into partnerships so large and strong that the HMOs couldn't afford to exclude them. For example:

The primary purpose, at least as I see it, there's an awful lot of talk about quality and integrated services and lower costs, [but] to me the primary purpose is that you're gathering together a mass to deal with managed care. It's economic to me. [CEO, suburban community hospital]

Economics (and survival) was closely linked to preservation of mission. For example, trustees were concerned with the continued provision of health care for the surrounding community or for a particular segment of the community (such as poor people), or with the delivery of certain kinds of specialty services. According to the CEO of a small and struggling urban hospital:

Since we faced, [and] some would argue continue to face, issues of survival as an institution, that was clearly on the top of the list. Which partner has the strongest commitment to [our neighborhood]? And would allow us—better, help us—to adhere to that mission. [CEO, urban community hospital]

Very few trustees spoke of affiliation arrangements as a means to improve quality of care, and just a few expressed the hope that quality would not be diminished by partnering. Those that focused on improved quality were primarily (but not exclusively) from one institution, a highly prestigious academic medical center:

One of the things that has been put up front in terms of this merger is that yes, we do want to affect savings; yes, we do want to have a better bottom line. But the real goal is to be the best quality delivery system. So quality is really way out in front. Our conviction is that quality will bring us financial success—people will pay for the best medical care, we believe. [Chair, academic medical center]

This institution has been building a network of affiliated hospitals, a strategy that was also described in terms of quality, in that the care provided in smaller hospitals in the network would be enhanced by the affiliation with the academic medical center. "People generally think a network is to bring people in," the CEO told us, "but it is also a means for disseminating quality services to a broader area."

Arrangements from Weakness

Among both our New York and conversion samples, there were certain hospitals for which partnering was essentially an act of desperation, seen as the only means of sustaining an institution that would otherwise be forced to close. At a hospital that was in New York State's Distressed Hospital Pool,[6] the new CEO explained, "bankruptcy was staring us in the face," and bills had gone unpaid for more than a year. Finally, New York State mandated a partnering arrangement, in which substantial control of the hospital was given to a neighboring hospital.

Three of the hospitals in the conversion sample had very severe financial problems, including large debt and little opportunity to overcome it. These problems had resulted from changing health care economics and market issues, such as the outside purchase of physician practices and the diversion of patients from suburban community hospitals to urban teaching hospitals—generally combined with some historical factors and poor administrative choices. In addition, these hospitals all had severe governance problems. Two individuals described the atmospherics of governance at their hospital, a hospital that considered, but decided against, selling to a for-profit company:

> In our situation, the trustees chose a banker to run the place. He was the chairman of the board before. He was fired as a banker, laid off, so they told him why go look for another bank, just come and run the hospital. He didn't know [anything] about the hospital. And the club continued. Finances became a big issue, and the physicians basically walked out on the board in a vote of no confidence. There were several votes of no confidence. The hospital was crashing down. . . . We had to move the hospital twice; it was a nightmare. [Trustee, urban community hospital]

> What happened here is we had an old-boy network. It had been in place for thirty to thirty-five years. A small clique was running the place and literally running it into the ground. [CEO, urban community hospital]

A second hospital that considered sale to a for-profit was $102 million in debt with revenues of $170 million and was in danger of defaulting on its loans. Operating rooms at one of its two campuses had not been renovated for twenty years; overall, $30–40 million dollars in capital improvements were needed. There had been several votes of no confidence by the physicians. Problems were primarily attributed to an incompetent CEO (now replaced) and an earlier two-hospital merger that had failed to achieve meaningful integration. One trustee described it this way:

> The merger that originally blended the campuses has never, ever, ever worked well. As time went on, we saw two camps developing who were really stuck in their own cultures and worked against one another. . . . By the time we came to do the joint venture, 95 percent of our primary care physician [practices] were owned by competing organizations. And the more established physicians worked at destroying any ability to recruit younger primary care physicians into the area. So we saw ourselves in a financially compromised position. [Trustee, suburban conversion hospital]

Furthermore (in the words of a trustee), the region has "too many beds, too many local institutions and everyone is trying to hold onto their organization. No trustee wants to be the one to shut the door."

A third hospital in our conversion sample (a specialty hospital that eventually declared bankruptcy) was in default of its bonds and had insufficient funds to meet payroll for the coming month. Revenues were covering just half of costs, and the services the hospital was providing could have easily been accommodated by competing institutions. According to the former CEO, the hospital, as it was operating, was no longer needed.

Arrangements from Strength

In contrast to those described above, there were certain hospitals that partnered relatively early on, while still financially strong. Surprisingly, two of the conversion hospitals, one that was sold and one that reorganized as a for-profit, had strong balance sheets and were acting in anticipation of what they felt was likely to occur in three, or even five years.[7] One of these was a specialty hospital. The trustees at this hospital believed that their institution had a distinctive approach to patient care but that its ability to function as an independent specialty hospital was threatened by marketplace factors. Similar to other institutions in our sample, this hospital needed a way to make itself larger. Local acute care hospitals sought to have the specialty hospital partner with them, but the trustees of the specialty hospital feared their institution would actually be taken over and possibly used for another purpose. Instead, as described in more detail below, they decided to reorganize as a for-profit to enhance the hospital's ability to grow via mergers and acquisitions of similar hospitals in other states.

The second of these two financially strong conversion institutions was owned by a university. For some time, the hospital had been a "cash cow" for the university, providing funds that the university was able to use for medical education and training purposes. However, in contrast to their neighboring institutions, which had partnered early on, this hospital lacked affiliate organizations for tertiary care referrals, and projections of their financial trend lines indicated that the hospital would generate revenue for just two more years. The third year, they would break even, and thereafter the university would have to subsidize the hospital. The trustees of the hospital saw its mission primarily in educational terms: to support the training of doctors and other health care professionals. And they feared that if the hospital's contribution to the university disappeared, its educational goals would be threatened. They decided to sell the hospital and use the proceeds for an endowment to support their medical education programs.

PARTNERING PROCESSES

The management and/or boards at virtually all hospitals that considered partnering made serious efforts to educate trustees on the subject, and on changes in health care more generally, by bringing in consultants and disseminating printed information. At the majority of hospitals, trustees went through a very careful and time-consuming planning process, which included reviews of revenue trend lines; creation of ad hoc committees; specification of criteria that a partner or partnering arrangement would have to meet; and discussions with a number of potential partners (as many as eight)—discussions that included trustees, administrative staff, and consultants.

At a small number of hospitals, substantial institutional changes were made in preparation for partnering, including internal restructuring and streamlining of the hospital and/or board (for "fast decisions and fast votes")—even selection of a new CEO, whose job was to make the hospital attractive to suitors and to then negotiate with them. Where sale to a for-profit was an option, the process usually included the hiring of legal and financial consultants, development of an RFP, and visits to other hospitals owned by potential purchasers. One hospital chartered a plane—"it was cheaper that way"—and took board members, community members, employees, and physicians to visit a distant hospital owned by a corporate bidder.

All the partnering arrangements took months to finalize. Some had taken years (one merger was first contemplated eighty years before, but that is a different story), with failed attempts sometimes preceding the successful one. A few institutions had switched from one affiliation arrangement to another, as they witnessed the adverse results of their first selection; as one trustee described the situation, "Whatever was going on there, we weren't getting what we needed" [trustee, urban teaching hospital]. In some cases, trustees of the smaller partners were disappointed by the inadequate system-building capacity of the larger institution or by the latter's lack of commitment (generally financial):

> We were providing [the partner hospital] with referrals, and certainly [their] medical school was thrilled with the hospital relationship. But it was static. [They were] not moving with the times. They have apparently, for whatever reason, been somewhat insulated from the changes in the last few years and have made much lesser strides in adapting to the changed hospital situation. [We have] no cushion. We are not in a position to let any time go by in adjusting to what's going on. [Trustee, urban teaching hospital]

In other cases, trustees of the smaller partner began to fear that the dominant partner had plans for their institution that ran counter to their interests (e.g., limiting the type of services provided), their conception of community interests, or the original agreements. According to the former chair of a small and struggling urban hospital: "[Our first partner] was leading us into being a strictly ambulatory care center, when we wanted to be as much a community hospital as possible. The [surrounding minority] community relies on us tremendously."

A trustee from a hospital in our conversion sample was similarly disappointed with his hospital's original partner:

> When [a nearby nonprofit] wanted to take us to create a system, they did sell us a vision. But the reality is that they looked back after a while, and they felt their chauvinistic thing is that they have to develop [their own hospital] and not here. And they denied what they promised, and they started basically undermining our community services for their financial benefit. And once that was clear, we just stood firm for our community. And we told them that's what you promised, that's what we want. And they said you have no options. And well, we'll find out whether we have an option or not. And we broke up. Now, we may have very well not found an option. And we may have very well gone back on bended knees and be closed. But that's where all the education of the board, and the cohesiveness, and commitment to the community and where a clear mission in their mind of what their role versus what their role isn't came into play. And they decided that if that's real, we have to know it, and if it's not we have to know. We came to the conclusion that we're going to have to do a public RFP. And of course the same hospital came back willing to pay $40 million to get us. [Trustee, suburban hospital]

PARTNERING CRITERIA

An essential part of the process toward partnering was the establishment of criteria for what the arrangement would entail. In our sample, individual institutions and trustees used a number of different criteria for selecting partners. In our New York–area sample, these most commonly included mission, similarity of mission, or the continuation thereof (seven hospitals). Other important criteria were a governance structure that allowed maximum autonomy for their institution (four hospitals), geographic proximity (three hospitals), complementarity in terms of location and clinical services (two hospitals), equality of institutions (with an expectation that agreements will be implemented in that spirit) (two hospitals), the potential for expansion of services or service area (two hospitals), similarity of culture (two hospitals), strength of network (two hospitals), and quality of medical education (two hospitals). Trustees described their criteria for partnering as follows:

> There had to be an identity of interests and health care goals. . . . There had to be an understanding by [the sponsoring organization] that it was incredibly important to the hospital to retain community control and identity, and it had to be translated into the actual sponsorship agreement. [Trustee, community hospital]

> High-quality teaching and willingness to bring [our physicians] in, to give them the titles they are entitled to, and to treat them as equals. [Trustee, urban teaching hospital]

Hospitals in the conversion sample, most of which went through the development of a formal RFP, had particularly clear criteria for acceptable deals and partners. These included community, mission, and governance concerns; minimum levels of uncompensated care; board representation; retirement of the debt and/or setting aside funds for a foundation or endowment; guarantees regarding a period of time that the hospital would remain open; guarantees regarding the delivery of particular services, such as emergency room services and services related to the hospital's traditional mission and orientation (be it teaching, specialty care, or religious); and in the case of a Catholic hospital, adherence to the religious directives of the Catholic Church.

With the exception of the hospital that reorganized as a for-profit company, none of the hospitals in the conversion sample was specifically seeking to become for-profit. All considered—and, in theory, favored—other possibilities, primarily partnering with nearby nonprofit hospitals or systems. Yet they generally came into "the mating game" late, after most of their competitors were part of some type of alliance or system. One trustee likened his hospital's situation to a game of musical chairs, "and we were the ones left standing." According to a trustee whose board eventually sold its hospital to a for-profit company:

> When we first decided that we were going to seek a partner, we almost certainly would have thought that that would have been one of the major nonprofits. . . .

I can remember sitting down in a preliminary initial conversation with some people from Columbia and I can remember in my own mind thinking, "Why are we leading these people on?—we're just not going to go in that direction." It was inconceivable to me that we would end up partnering with a for-profit because I didn't understand for-profit and I didn't understand what the ultimate differences might be. So, I'd say that we sort of entered into the conversations that we had with the for-profit potential partners with the idea being that they would give us leverage in negotiating with the nonprofit partners that we would eventually end up getting together with. [Trustee, suburban conversion hospital]

Trustees we interviewed considered the sale option only after other attempted partnerships—partnerships that were short of a sale—proved unsuccessful:

We spent the year negotiating with four potential partners. The truth is I never wanted to sell to a for-profit, for a lot of different reasons. . . . When [Hospital M, a Catholic hospital] sold to Columbia/HCA there was a message. To be honest, I didn't want a Jewish hospital to be the first to sell to a for-profit. Once the Sisters [of Hospital M] sold—that possibility, of seeing what opportunities might exist, was one we had to pursue, so we pursued it. If I had my druthers, I would have preferred a merger with [Hospital N, a major local nonprofit], and we spent a year negotiating with them. Unfortunately, there were some key issues we couldn't resolve when we got down to the moment of truth. . . . [The for-profit] was the last entry and their offer was the best, and they met the criteria we'd established as an executive committee as to what we want in a partner. [Chair, urban teaching hospital]

STAKEHOLDER INPUT

Trustees from the New York–area sample generally mentioned little input or concern with their partnering decisions from the community, hospital staff, or others. An important exception was a nonsectarian hospital that chose to merge with a Catholic hospital. Residents of the local community wanted to be sure that the merger would not reduce access to reproductive health services, and the merger was arranged in such a way that existing services were maintained. By contrast, hospitals in the conversion sample generally received a great deal of input into their decisions. Two hospitals in the conversion sample (one that decided to sell to a for-profit and one that did not) *chose* to have a very public decision-making process. At the hospital that decided against conversion, trustees walked the hospital floors asking staff for their preferences; public presentations and visits to hospitals of the bidders were arranged; and employees were invited to speak at the board meeting where the decision would be made. These employees, in fact, swayed the highly influential vote of the CEO. At this hospital, the input of all stakeholders was considered essential to making the proper decision. In contrast, at the hospital that did convert to for-profit status, the emphasis was on providing information to those concerned about the hospital, so they would understand and accept the reasoning behind whatever decision was made—as they apparently did.

Whether by design (as in the two cases above) or not, sales to for-profit purchasers generally received a significant amount of public scrutiny, including numerous press accounts, open meetings, and reviews by the state attorney general. Depending on the institution, hospital physicians and staff, community advocates, and religious leaders all had opinions that could not be ignored. With the exception of the first groups, who generally favored the option that seemed most likely to guarantee their jobs (and salaries), most other parties were opposed to for-profit health care, due to concerns about charity care, quality, local control, and the payment of health care dollars to stockholders.

Consequently, trustees considering sale to a for-profit generally knew they were risking public disapproval. "It was very difficult," said one trustee whose hospital sold to a for-profit, "difficult because it made us pariahs. We took a lot of abuse for this." Only one of the trustees interviewed admitted that public opinion affected his vote, and some voted boldly against very powerful interests, including local and nationally prominent religious leaders. Still, it was sometimes apparent that trustees were influenced by the belief that a specific and very visible decision would be publicly criticized, particularly where board members saw themselves as representative of that public. At one hospital, where trustees made a last-minute decision not to sell to a for-profit, despite believing that this option had substantial net economic advantages, it was likely that at least some trustees were influenced by public sentiment.

In a unique case, a specialty hospital was negotiating a merger with a neighboring acute care hospital. The trustees and the CEO felt that such an agreement would benefit both institutions. The specialty hospital had a good facility but insufficient patients. The neighboring hospital had patients but was in need of a new facility. Yet the agreement was destroyed, according to those interviewed, by physicians who feared a merger would result in a reduction of their generous salary levels to those at the potential partner institution. The physicians threatened to place an advertisement in the local newspaper exposing purported conflicts of interest of board members. The board then resigned; shortly thereafter the CEO resigned, and partnering negotiations ended.

Agreements Reached: The New York–Area Sample

With all the possible choices and conflicting concerns, partnering represents a complex set of decisions for trustees. Not surprisingly, some reported considerable uncertainty and difficulty in assessing their choices. For example, one trustee explained how his hospital significantly enlarged its catchment area via its choice of partners, operating under the assumption that coverage of a wide area would help them to negotiate with managed care companies, "But it is a fluid situation and hard to prove." He said they had also considered joining with a nearby institution with the idea of achieving cost savings rather than geographic distribution—which also would have made sense. Basically, he commented, with so much uncertainty in health care, "you can rationalize any decision you make." Other trustees expressed concern about the conditions under which they were making decisions that affected the very core of their hospital's identity, currently and in the future:

> You can learn a certain amount [about health care delivery], but to some extent you have to take on faith that mingling, merging of institutions is something that is an intelligent response to the system as it is changing. Is it a crap shoot? A little bit. Nobody is really sure down the road how this is going to play out. Is it important for us to [purchase Hospital X] for that reason, yeah. But it's a little bit like you weigh the pros and cons and then you do the best you can. [Trustee, academic medical center]

> We are dealing with shifting sands, and anybody that tells me they really understand what is going on I think is deluding him- or herself. [Trustee, urban teaching hospital]

Yet most of the trustees we interviewed expressed comfort with their partnering decisions, which were, after all, quite recent. For the New York–area sample, most reservations focused on governance and trade-offs between the perceived benefits of arrangements and their price—which was always the loss or dilution of control:

> In the euphoria resulting from receiving financial assistance, it is easy to lose sight of the Faustian transaction taking place. . . . Trustees must be sure that changing the structure in this way services their purpose. They lose the right to call the shots, but the financial support does allow them to fulfill their mission. [Trustee, urban community hospital]

Most concerns focused on control in the long term, because agreements often had conditions regarding governance that would *gradually* erode autonomy or that held for a limited number of years. For example—as is typical of four hospitals in the sample—Hospital A is now a sponsored hospital within a large system. They have 3 (out of 120) representatives on the system board. The system has 3 (out of 25) members on the hospital board. The system approves any new appointments to the hospital board, and after nine years it can replace any of the currently standing members. The system can also double the size of the board if it chooses to, thereby diminishing the authority of the original trustees. But it has not done so to date.

Hospital B is also a sponsored hospital. It is in a different, equally large system, and board representation and control are similar to those described for Hospital A. At both hospitals, any new board members selected by the system must come from the community surrounding the hospital. Also similar to Hospital A, the board of Hospital B has significant autonomy in hiring and firing the CEO, approving the hospital's budget, and internal operations. But the system has certain reserved powers, which have not yet been invoked, regarding divestiture of real property and major assets, the sale or lease of the hospital, and major changes to its bylaws.

Some trustees of hospitals that had entered into sponsorship arrangements worried about their institution's vulnerability to changes in management at the dominant institution and about the possibility that agreements that had been reached might be interpreted differently when the cast of characters changes. But these long-term concerns were generally muted because of their belief that their institutions were valuable to the dominant institutions, because the need to attend to immediate survival issues had been so pressing, or because of the health care benefits that they saw for their community. Two trustees at an urban teaching hospital explained:

> If we ever get fat and complacent, where the main issue of the board meeting is having dinner together with our good fellows . . . we ought to be kicked off. We're not going to kick ourselves off. [The system board] will be able to do that. . . . But it is within their interest to have a strong board with [community] leaders on it. So as long as our board is strong (and they will try to help us make it stronger) if we have a problem, they're going to deal with us at arm's length. [Trustee, urban teaching hospital]

> I'm sure if you talked to board members at [our hospital], there are some who would flair up on the issue of losing control. I am trying to stay focused on the delivery of class health care to a large area of [the community] that is not otherwise being served. . . . I don't want to sound like somebody who is ready to just give up and walk away, but I think that we must think not about our board's control. [We] must think about the broad picture of what's happening in the city and what's happening in the delivery of health care. . . . I feel a commitment to what the institution does. I don't feel such a commitment to how it does it, in corporate structure terms. [Trustee, urban teaching hospital]

This trustee felt she could be somewhat objective because she had served on the board for just six years and was not yet "an insider," whose primary allegiance was to the institution itself. A small number of other trustees also felt that their lack of a strong allegiance to their particular institutions helped them to accomplish the most advantageous arrangements for the institution and the community, in this case, a full-asset merger. The board chair of an academic medical center mentioned that he and the chair of the hospital with which they merged could have just as easily been in the opposite positions, being the sort of "corporate guys around town" that hospitals like to have on their boards. He went on to observe that

> it's a lovely thing when somebody has a very warm and fuzzy identity with the hospital and it goes back over generations. But it also creates some myopia in terms of where you were and what you're about. And I honestly believe that being somewhat dispassionate although very involved with our respective hospitals enabled us to get over some of the hooks that precluded other hospitals from doing the same thing. [Chair, academic medical center]

Five hospitals in the New York–area sample had chosen something akin to a merger: an actual full-asset merger, a joint venture, or the creation of a holding company. Mergers were seen as allowing institutions to preserve and even extend their mission, by expanding their catchment area and enhancing their bargaining position with respect to managed care organizations:

> And here is [our hospital], a very successful, financially strong, diversified, grow-ing, geographically dispersed health care delivery system: Do we go it alone? And having decided that for a whole variety of reasons . . . [that] it was important for us to go beyond just [our hospital] and basically to give up our autonomy and to put it into the hands of a holding company so we could affect the partnership with [Hospital C] and attract others to join us as well. . . . Basically what [our hospital] has done is put its fate into the hands of a holding company that it does not control. And we did it because we felt that this was in the interest of all the institutions that would come to join us. [Chair, urban teaching hospital]

Merger-like arrangements were used where there were two institutions of similar strength and by smaller institutions that were hoping to avoid "being swallowed up." Although the combined or holding company board may have greater powers (with respect to the individual hospital boards) than in a spon-sorship arrangement, the constituent hospitals—generally no more than three—have far greater representation on that newly created board than in the sponsorship situation.

THE CONVERSION SAMPLE: THE FOR-PROFIT OPTION

Of the six hospitals in the conversion sample, three decided to sell, one reorga-nized as a for-profit, and two decided not to sell—although at one of these a final affiliation arrangement was not agreed upon at the time of our interviews.

Some trustees who came to favor a for-profit option feared that merging with a nearby nonprofit would essentially mean giving their hospital away—possibly to a hospital that was not necessarily stronger, in financial terms, than theirs. One trustee of an urban teaching hospital explained: "In essence, they wanted us to just give them the keys and say we're partners. But we would be the minority partner."

At sample institutions in which negotiations with nonprofits broke down, the reasons generally centered on concerns about inadequate board representation, the lack of funds for a foundation such as would be created in a for-profit sale, and a fear that the nonprofit into which they would merge would close the hospital once they had control of it.

Once the nonprofit options were seen as infeasible, many trustees described having to overcome their biases against for-profit health care, as well as their concerns about community perceptions. One CEO noted with amusement that for a board whose members primarily worked in the for-profit sector, their expressed lack of trust in for-profit health care was surprising. But not everyone was alarmed by the for-profit option. One trustee explained that they were always "running a tight ship," "doing a good job with the business." He commented that for-profits look at the bottom line and that keeps them disciplined, but with the changes in health care, nonprofits must do the same. Others expressed similar views:

> For-profit/not-for-profit was not an issue with our employees, with the community. Because the community was looking at what are these guys going to do to save our hospital. [CEO, urban community hospital]

> [The for-profit company] is a bottom-line-accountable organization. But the reality is so is every other nonprofit health care provider. When I was heading up a citizens organization here, we did a study on health care for the medically indigent . . . charity care, give me a break, these are not people who are looking to take care of poor folk. The little nuns that did it because that was their mission from God don't do that anymore. And the guys running these hospitals are not in the business of taking care of poor folks. They haven't been for some long time. As soon as the belt started tightening, it went through the food chain. [Trustee, conversion hospital]

At three institutions that sold to for-profits, trustees emphasized innovative aspects of their decision, seeing themselves as leaders in the field. The CEO of the specialty hospital that converted to for-profit status commented that he had some ten years until retirement. In this relatively brief time, he did not want to be a "bystander or a pawn." He saw himself as a mover and wanted to be part of moving his institution in a direction that would benefit the whole field.

In every case where the for-profit option was chosen, definite advantages were cited. At one hospital, the for-profit offered $300 million compared with the nonprofit's $200 million, equal (rather than minority) representation on the hospital's post-sale board, and greater guarantees regarding charity care and continuation of the hospital's teaching mission. The for-profit, in fact, met all the board's conditions for sale, including conditions that the nonprofit suitors did not meet. One trustee described the arrangement as follows:

> We built into that all the safeguards that the folks like me really struggled greatly with. I mean the financial folks can struggle with finances but the rest of us struggle with the rest of it. And the rest of it included issues related to the church, issues related to charity care and mission, issues related to the medical students. [Trustee, urban conversion hospital]

The financial aspects of the deals were also important, in part, as tangible evidence of the commitment of the purchaser:

> We felt that if somebody was actually going to sit down and write a check, in this case a check for about $80 million, that that represented a very, very serious commitment. They had to make the hospital successful. Otherwise they would have made a very bad investment. . . . It was in their self-interest to make the facility work. It wasn't in their self-interest to just pick off the cream from the top or divert patients to another facility or acquire the medical practices, which is one of the things that we thought could happen [if we merged] with the downtown nonprofit. [Trustee, conversion hospital]

Financial aspects were also important for the foundation or endowment they would support. Foundations were started with tens of millions of dollars and—in our sample—were controlled by those same board members who served on the hospital board. As the trustees viewed it, the foundations, once established, would allow them to continue to serve the institution's health care mission, albeit beyond the hospital walls.

Unique in our sample was a specialty hospital (described above) that reorganized itself into a for-profit organization. Trustees at the institution felt that to preserve the hospital's mission, it would need to get bigger and that the most natural combination would be with similar specialty hospitals in other states. Merging with these hospitals, however, would dilute their control over the resulting combined entity, perhaps also diluting their institution's distinctive approaches to patient care. Thus, they wished to grow by acquisition, which would require access to capital. They rejected the idea of using debt for this purpose. Instead, they chose to reorganize, putting the hospital into a for-profit organization, with 100 percent of the stock owned by their existing foundation, which supports research, education, and charity care.[8] Either this stock, or stock from subsequent offerings, could be used as the currency with which to acquire other hospitals. (Not surprisingly, this board of trustees had strong representation from the investment banking world.) A secondary benefit of this arrangement was mentioned by several trustees we interviewed: Stock options could be offered to employees, increasing their incentives to perform and enhancing the organization's ability to attract top managerial talent. The justification given by the CEO was similar to what we heard from trustees:

> If you strip out those things that are appreciated and reimbursed in the marketplace from the others, namely, research and education, that are not appreciated and therefore not reimbursed then what you've got, theoretically, is a well-functioning, lean, good provider, and then you've got value over here that can be used for the advancement of the field. [CEO, specialty hospital]

An implication of this arrangement is that the two organizations—the for-profit hospital and its nonprofit parent foundation—would be operated in a mutually beneficial way. The foundation would not expect to receive dividends, so that the hospital could accumulate assets to further its expansion plans. The object of the foundation's research, education, and charity care activities would primarily be the hospital and the specialty care it provides. The trustees we interviewed took pains to explain that the arrangement had been closely scrutinized by the state attorney general's office and, despite the fact that the boards had key interlocking members, it had passed muster. Several mentioned steps that had been taken to minimize conflict of interest, including an explicit decision regarding whether trustees who had made the reorganization decision could benefit from the receipt of stock options.

This case raises important issues regarding the responsibilities of trustees. The trustees we interviewed all argued that this arrangement was the best way to assure the pursuit of their institution's mission—but the mission and economic interests of a nonprofit foundation are not generally so closely tied to the well-being of a single for-profit firm. Whatever the legalities of the arrangement, the case raises an important issue regarding the ethical responsibilities of trustees. Are there limits to the financial options that a nonprofit board might consider in furthering their organization's mission?

THE NONPROFIT OPTION

As was mentioned above, just two of the six hospitals in our conversion sample remained nonprofits. At one, the final partnering arrangements have not yet been decided upon. The second hospital is the only one in the sample that purposely chose the nonprofit over for-profit option. After months of reviews of alternatives, a public meeting, and extensive consultation with doctors and hospital employees, the trustees and the CEO told us that their decisions as

individuals and as a board were made at the final moment, at the end of a
seven-hour meeting, lasting past midnight:

> We'd go around the room and ask everyone to make their comments. This was
> what I would call an open conscious program in which we made everybody talk.
> Nobody could escape without making comments on the different areas. Because
> we wanted to make sure, whatever we did, I mean we understood the gravity—if
> you will the severity of the decision. [CEO, suburban community hospital]

According to both the CEO and trustees interviewed, the vote could have
easily gone either way. A for-profit company was offering to set up a $22 mil-
lion foundation. This option was overwhelmingly preferred by the employees,
who feared the nonprofit system that sought to acquire them via merger would
consolidate and eventually close them down. Local politicians and health advocates favored the nonprofit system, believing it would be more responsive to
regulatory issues. For most trustees interviewed, as well as the CEO, an important factor was that the for-profit did not have any managed care contracts in
the state, which raised a question about the hospital's future if that option was
chosen. One trustee said that he voted the way he felt a "person living in the
community" would have, despite the fact that he thought that person would
have been wrong. Another considered the impact of the alternatives on a
neighboring hospital:

> [The neighboring hospital] is only five miles away, and their trust fund, and their
> buildings, and their equipment, and so on and so forth belong to the community
> just like I do. And [if we were] to get a for-profit to compete with them, they
> might waste 30, 40, 60 million, or even worse and close down. I felt that I am a
> trustee of community resources and that includes [the neighboring hospital]. I
> felt very strongly that [that hospital] is my community wealth and I don't want
> that destroyed. That weighed very heavy on my heart. [Trustee, suburban com-
> munity hospital]

It is also important to note how much the nonprofit system offered in
response to its fear of the for-profit:

> We met with [the nonprofit] the day before. We put this outlandish demand on
> the table. We want 50 percent of the board. [Our CEO] does not report to [the
> existing CEO], he becomes a member of the board . . . and will report to the
> board. Both board chairmen will be co-chairman, until six months after we sign
> this deal. And then we'll make a decision about the board chairman. . . . We
> could have asked for their wives and children. I'm not kidding. It was amazing.
> They were afraid of [the for-profit firm] coming in and [there] being competition
> in the marketplace. [CEO, suburban community hospital][9]

However, the one thing that was not demanded or received was payment for the hospital, so the opportunity to create a community foundation from the hospital's assets was lost.

PARTNERS: MAKING IT WORK

Although the creation of partnering arrangements was difficult and time consuming for trustees, the work did not end once the agreements were made. After partnership arrangements were agreed upon, trustees often faced problems of melding of cultures, integrating medical staffs, realizing the efficiencies that were part of the rationale for the deal—it was hoped, in the opinion of the trustees interviewed, without layoffs—and determining priorities for individual hospitals and the system as a whole. Partners do not necessarily come together prepared to work productively through these issues:

Even though we're now part of the system . . . make no mistake. To be part of the system doesn't mean they don't steal [patients] from us. I mean they take care of themselves first, which is understandable. [CEO, suburban community hospital]

Culturally, we have to think differently because [Hospital A] was one thing, [Hospital B] another, and we were another. And now it's all sort of coming together and we're trying to find the efficiencies economically in running these as one, and we need to find how to live culturally with a more diverse eclectic group of people. And that takes a little bit of a struggle, I guess. It doesn't just happen. [Trustee, urban teaching hospital]

Smaller partners must adjust to the fact that they can no longer make all the decisions themselves. To some extent, they no longer control their own fate. Trustees at the larger partners, who previously had allegiance (sometimes over generations) to a single institution, now must consider the interests of all the partners on a supposedly site-blind basis. As one trustee explained:

Our board chair has taken the position that we are a hospital network as opposed to a New York City hospital, and the revenue generated by the network is just as important as the revenue generated by the catchment area of [this hospital]. And as a board, we have a responsibility to each and not just to what we might think of as our own. [Trustee, academic medical center]

At some institutions, trustees believe that efficiencies and cost savings have occurred. One teaching hospital was reported to have achieved $33 million in savings in just over a year through the consolidation of information systems, purchasing, human resources, food service, and finance. At other institutions, additional benefits were claimed, including access to improved administrators and trustees (through the health care systems), information systems, and capital.

For the hospitals in our conversion sample, the future is already less clear. The specialty hospital that converted to for-profit status has not yet convinced others to join it. According to the CEO, "It is harder to actually pull off than it was to conceptualize. . . . No one wants to be the first to jump in." Two hospitals in the conversion sample were purchased by companies that subsequently had serious financial problems of their own (one, in fact, declared bankruptcy) and were therefore unable to fulfill promises made. One of these hospitals has been sold to another for-profit company, and the trustees are cautiously optimistic that conditions of the original sale will now be fulfilled. As was mentioned above, one institution—the one whose board resigned under pressure from the medical staff—has not yet developed an affiliation with other organizations. The other two (one that sold to a for-profit company and one that did not) are satisfied with the arrangements they made, feeling that they are working as well as or better than anticipated.

CONCLUSION

The long-term outcome of the partnering and conversions described here is, of course, still to be determined. We did find that trustees across institutions believe that the market demands that hospitals be larger and have more negotiating power, or their survival will be threatened. And they have obviously been acting on that belief. Yet the descriptions we heard regarding past affiliation arrangements that eventually dissolved or that resulted in worsened financial status—even closure—show that partnering is not a panacea for hospital ills or worries. If our sample is at all representative, it is likely that some of these arrangements will prove beneficial and some will not.

In making their partnering decisions, trustees in both our New York–area and conversion samples had to face a number of difficult problems. They had to carefully balance concerns about fidelity to mission, autonomy, commitment to community, short-term financial needs, and the potential for long-term survival. In doing so, they may have had to consider the proper responsibility of a trustee: Was their responsibility to represent their own best judgment or to represent the wishes (even if misguided) of the community? Were they there to ensure the survival of the hospital as an institution or to ensure access to health care in the community? In fact, there was little evidence that trustees considered "community" separate from the hospital. At no hospital did trustees seriously consider closing, despite their recognition of local overbedding. Similarly, there was no mention of services being reduced. Furthermore, few trustees seem to seriously consider the impact of their decisions on nearby hospitals.

Trustees in the conversion sample clearly faced the most difficult of decisions. Although they might have felt that the profit motive is antithetical to the inherent purpose of a hospital, they could not help but notice that for-profits may have significantly more to offer a struggling hospital and its community. Yet sale (generally to national firms based far from the site of the hospital) and the creation of a foundation involves a fundamental transformation in the asset that they held in trust, a transformation that may not be justifiable in all cases.

Options considered by hospitals in the New York area had to do with the benefits of joining with one or another local institution or system, and the benefits of one or another type of partnering arrangement, including acquisition of other institutions, merger, and joining a network (while retaining various degrees of autonomy). Virtually all these arrangements involved some change in governance and institutional autonomy—which in turn led to concerns about preservation of institutional ethos, community service roles, and survival (i.e., "Are they partnering with us just to close us down?"). For both samples, all decisions took place within an environment of great uncertainty and constant change.

In developing partnering and affiliation agreements, trustees had to separate out and balance the component parts of what they hold in trust: the hospital as an institution, health care or research and education as a mission that might be pursued in different ways, and the sometimes diverse communities the hospital serves. Our research highlights the difficulty of this task, the enormous responsibility trustees have voluntarily accepted, as well as the broad range of skills, resources, and concerns they bring to this process.

NOTES

1. B. Japsen, "An Off Year for Consolidation," *Modern Healthcare* 28, no. 2 (1998): 40–48.

2. S. L. Isaacs, D. F. Beatrice, and W. Carr, "Health Care Conversion Foundations: A Status Report," *Health Affairs* 16, no. 6 (1997): 228–36; Tami Mark, *The Community Impact of For-Profit Hospital Conversions* (Millwood, Va.: Center for Health Affairs, Project Hope, 1997).

3. D. Bellandi, "Healthcare Mergers, Acquisitions Plunge," *Modern Healthcare* 29, no. 31 (1999): 20.

4. This category is underrepresented in our sample due to a high number of refusals to participate.

5. Because of the press that surrounded most of these cases, we have chosen to limit the amount of descriptive information provided.

6. Four hospitals in our sample were members of this pool, which provides funding to financially distressed hospitals across New York State.

7. Nationally, hospitals that convert to for-profit status are more financially precarious and have significantly lower profit margins and patient volume, as compared with other hospitals (Mark, *Community Impact*, viii, x).

8. The foundation was established as a supporting organization rather than as a private foundation, giving it an ongoing obligation to raise public support and relieving it of requirements that apply to private foundations.

9. Trustees from small hospitals in our New York sample expressed similar sentiments. They felt they got advantageous deals from more powerful neighboring institutions, because those latter institutions feared that the small hospital would partner with someone else and become a stronger competitor.

11

FITTING BOARD INFORMATION TO BOARD FUNCTION

Anthony R. Kovner

Governance is the system for making important decisions, and the board is that part of the organization under law that designs or partic-ipates in this system.[1] Members of the board are called trustees or directors. Not-for-profit boards lack the accountability that for-profit boards have to shareholders, and governmental legislative branches have to voters.

Questions have been raised regarding the accountability and performance of boards of directors of not-for-profit health care organizations, and regarding the poor quality of the information they receive to carry out board functions.[2] According to a recent Ernst & Young survey of 2,079 hospitals and 126 health systems, the information that hospital and health system boards routinely review "is a poorly examined aspect of hospital governance."[3]

The basic argument that I wish to make is that governing boards require information to carry out their functions, and most hospital boards with which I am familiar do not get this required information in user-friendly form. First, I review the literature that pertains to this argument, and, second, I relate my own experience as a not-for-profit hospital board member for 16 years.

BACKGROUND

The environment facing health care organizations is changing rapidly;[4] more competition, increasingly managing more risk, and more demanding customers. Not-for-profit health care organizations are becoming larger and more complex, with frequent mergers attributable to a need to obtain sufficient bargaining power vis-à-vis managed care organizations, many of which are national, investor-owned large corporations.[5]

Although there is general agreement in the literature about not-for-profit board functions, there is a lack of consensus regarding critical functions and the recommended priorities among activities under each function.[6] Of course, critical functions and priorities among activities are expected to vary, by organization and circumstance.[7] Not everyone agrees with John Carver that boards, which under state law are owners of not-for-profit organizations, should actually function as owners.[8] There is general agreement that boards do guide long-range planning decisions, evaluate organizational and top management performance, and are often involved in fundraising. According to Shoshonna Sofaer and her colleagues, little is known about how nonprofit hospital and health system boards actually function, not to mention the relationship of these functions to organizational performance.[9]

William Bowen states that boards, whether for-profit or not-for-profit, serve six principal functions.[10] These are to (1) select, encourage, advise, evaluate and, if need be, replace the chief executive officer (CEO); (2) review and adapt long-term strategic directions and to approve specific objectives, financial and other; (3) monitor the performance of management; (4) ensure, to the extent possible, that the necessary resources, including human resources will be available to pursue the strategies and achieve the objectives; (5) ensure that the organization operates responsibly as well as effectively; and (6) nominate suitable candidates for election to the board, and to establish and carry out an effective system of governance at the board level, including evaluation of board governance. Consistent with Bowen, Carver specifies the principal functions of not-for-profit boards as to (1) guide long-range planning and (2) evaluate top management and current organizational performance. Dennis Pointer and Charles Ewell specify board responsibilities in terms of policy formulation and oversight; they also include decision making.[11] They note that some smaller boards perform managerial work, as well as spending a lot of time and energy raising funds.

As not-for-profit boards increasingly become responsible for larger and more geographically spread out facilities and programs, this may affect the way the board functions. Pointer and his colleagues suggest that, increasingly, in large not-for-profit health care organizations, boards will be responsible for a more-or-less integrated network of organizations rather than a single institution.[12] This change and intensifying competition, as well, may increasingly strain current governance functions. Activities within these functions may also change. Pointer and his colleagues suggest that rather than making decisions about management actions, such as approval of construction plans, budget changes, physician privileges, and response to malpractice events, boards will be increasingly shaping and making complex strategic decisions, such as investment in recruitment of primary care physicians, clinical integration in merged or affiliated organizations, and investment in information technology and in radically improving quality and service to customers. Typically such strategic decisions require trade-offs and impose major risks to organizational survival and growth.

Pointer and his colleagues suggest that given changing circumstances, different board configurations should be considered to include the following: members no longer chosen to be representative of certain constituencies and stakeholders, insiders other than the CEO on the board, compensation for boards, different types of standing committees, unifying CEO and board chairperson roles, and professional full-time staffing.

As board membership, functions and structure change in such complex organizations, the information boards require to make effective decisions may be quite different from that required to function in smaller, simpler organizations facing more stable environments. Because of the risks and trade-offs involved nonprofit boards are forced to act more, as Carver proposes, as "corporate owners," for example, as the character and even survival of an organization are increasingly challenged by fast-breaking events, such as a state government's mandating of Medicaid managed care or a competitor's merging with a much larger institution.

ISSUES AND CONCERNS ABOUT GOVERNANCE INFORMATION

In examining the infrastructure of good decision-making processes at three leading large health care organizations, John Griffith and his colleagues suggest that boards cannot implement effective decision-making processes without information regarding stakeholders as well as their expectations and perceptions.[13] Little research, other than the Ernst & Young survey, has been done to document what kinds of information non-profit boards typically receive. For example, "information" is not even listed in the index of the most authoritative work on current hospital and health system governance by Pointer and Ewell. Nor is there anything in the published literature regarding best practices with regard to board information systems, and efforts of boards to get better information.

In their 1997 survey, consultants at Ernst & Young found that most boards surveyed obtained information on the following topics: operating statistics, budget performance, financial statement performance, capital planning, patient satisfaction surveys, mortality rates, employee attitude surveys, morbidity rates, and unscheduled readmissions. This leaves many gaps in areas such as provider and purchaser satisfaction and managed care performance, and there is also no indication in the Ernst & Young survey that patient satisfaction surveys, for example, were presented in a way that was particularly useful for board guidance of long-range strategic planning or to inform board evaluation of organizational performance, for example, in areas such as cardiac or cancer care.

J. E. Orlikoff and M. K. Totten identify the following nine common flaws in board information:[14]

- Reports and information do not flow from or support the explicitly defined role of the board on the issue.
- There are no guidelines regarding what information should be reported to the board or how it should be reported.
- Reports provide data, such as clinical indicators, but not information, such as trends or projections.
- Meeting minutes are used as a vehicle for providing information to the Board (e.g., the finance committee minutes are used as the financial report to the Board).
- Too much material is presented in the reports.
- Governance reports are simply management or medical staff information with a new title.
- Ineffective report formats blunt the Board's understanding of important information.
- Thick Board agenda packets are distributed to Board members so close to the scheduled meeting that there's no time to read all the material.
- Significant amounts of informational materials are routinely distributed to Board members for review at the Board meeting.

The Ernst & Young consultants recommended that at a minimum, a competitive health system should be able to measure the following: financial performance, patient satisfaction, purchaser satisfaction, provider satisfaction, clinical outcomes, and managed care performance. Ernst & Young did not seek information in their survey as to whether the boards surveyed received regular and routine information regarding how the organization appears to customers, physicians, market share and competitor information, and information about best clinical and management practices. Nor did they indicate that on a regular basis such board members receive explanations for variance between current hospital or health system operating performance and best service and management practices for similar organizations. Nor did they indicate that at many hospitals and health systems there is either regular monitoring of, or planned adaptation by the board with regard to the organization's mission, objectives, and strategy.

There is no evidence in the Ernst & Young survey, or anywhere else in the literature, that not-for-profit hospital and health system boards regularly get the information they need to carry out the functions they are supposed to perform as owners of or decision makers in these organizations.

MY EXPERIENCE AS A BOARD MEMBER

I believe that trustees have an ethical obligation to make sure that they receive materials that are adequate for them to carry out their functions. Those who have written about the functions of trustees describe these functions in differing terms. I believe there is some level of consensus around at least three basic functions: (1) evaluating top management, (2) managing the governance process, and (3) planning the longer-range future of the organization. Griffith describes the well-managed health care organization as pursuing results across four dimensions: access, technical quality, satisfaction, and cost.[15] Thus a well-managed board would presumably want information regarding hospital and health care system performance along these four dimensions.

Before describing my experience, I should provide a few facts about myself and the hospital on whose board I have been sitting. I am a sixty-five-year-old professor of health policy and management, whose academic specialty is not-for-profit governance. I have been a CEO of a community hospital, and I have consulted to a variety of nonprofit organizations, including hospitals, to improve their governance. The hospital, now medical center, on whose board I have sat, is large, not-for-profit, and urban, with a well-developed community service mission, owned by a church whose central headquarters are in another part of the country. From 1983 to 1996, and for many years before that, the hospital was managed by one CEO, who retired in 1996, and had one Board Chair, who remained chair as of 1999.

The period 1983–96. For the first thirteen years of my board service, I was dissatisfied with the information the board received at monthly meetings, but I did nothing about it. The information had been primarily financial, and it was often distributed only at the board meetings. The financial information had been very lengthy (between twenty and sixty pages), difficult to understand, and with no introductory memo explaining performance, variance, or reasons for variance. This was against the background of a hospital that was not losing money, with a very strong CEO and a very strong board chair. I shared my feelings of dissatisfaction with the chief operating officer and with other administrators but never with the CEO, who was on record with me as strongly opposed to a board that micromanages. Rather, the CEO saw the primary purpose of the board as supporting the CEO and, in general terms, evaluating his performance.

From 1996 to the present. The hospital was reorganized as a medical center. This meant that some previously owned facilities that had been operated separately now came under the board's supervision. The hospital board became the board for the medical center as well as the hospital. The subsidiaries retained their existing boards. They included a large nursing home, a large health maintenance organization (HMO), and other smaller facilities. Total revenues for the medical center were more than $250 million.

At a board meeting during the spring of 1997, I shared my concerns about information received by the board at a board meeting when the financials were being reviewed. One of the other board members asked me whether I could share with the others some "models of governance information systems." After the meeting, I went through my files and sent to her and to three other board leaders and the CEO the following materials: (1) an article "Information and the Effective Board," by Orlikoff and Totten,[16] (2) an article titled "Checking the Dashboard," by MacKaye,[17] (3) a spider diagram used by "Walke-Parke" Medical Center (fictional name) with 1993 targets, (4) results at the Massachusetts General Hospital on five key performance indicators,[18] and (5) R. S. Kaplan and D. P. Norton's balanced scorecard approach[19] (which focused on four dimensions: building an organizational consensus around vision and strategy, communicating and linking strategy up and down the organization and linking it to departmental and individual objectives, business planning to integrate business and financial plans, and feedback and learning). I wrote these individuals that I would greatly appreciate comments and questions. But I received none.

In January 1998, I wrote to the CEO, formerly the chief operating officer, to follow up, jotting down areas about which I as a board member would like to get better information. These included: the percentage of patients who were completely or very satisfied, physician satisfaction survey, net operating income, market share by main service lines, total donations received, uncompensated care, cost leadership, employee satisfaction, managed care enrollment, and accreditation performance. I said that I would like to discuss with him the areas he thought it was important to regularly inform the board on through indicators and those that he deemed unimportant. I followed up again with him a few weeks after writing him the memo, after which he informed me in his office that changing the information that the board regularly received "was a great idea but he had more important things to do." Subsequently, this CEO resigned, and he was replaced by an interim CEO, the medical center counsel.

After that, I enlisted the support of one of the senior hospital administrators, in charge of quality improvement, who together with the administrative resident volunteered to work with me on developing a draft of performance indicators that top management could regularly report to the board. We used the following criteria to develop the indicators: (1) we would not be limited to financial indicators, (2) we would rely on existing data, (3) we would go beyond the hospital and include indicators on nursing home and HMO performance, and (4) we would use indicators for which we could also develop standards of performance.

The proposed performance indicators are shown in table 11.1. Indicators were divided along four dimensions with four indicators for each dimension. The dimensions were as follows: financial, growth and development, quality, and customer satisfaction. For each indicator we developed a target and rationale and compared this with actual performance. Our report was presented to the Finance Committee in June 1999, but there was not sufficient time at that meeting to allow for significant discussion.

After the meeting, and not having heard anything from any of the board members, I wrote to the finance chair, asking his guidance as to how to proceed. I emphasized that what we had developed was a first step toward what we hoped would produce something genuinely useful for the board. As of this writing, I had not heard anything from him or from any of the other committee members.

Lessons Learned

What I believe I have learned from this experience, so far, is that changing the information that board members receive regularly may be a difficult process for a lone board member to accomplish. Such change may not be feasible until the board is "ready" and convinced that the benefits to be gained from the change outweigh the costs, that is, that the information will be used to change behavior rather than as an end in itself. Getting the board "ready" could have been facilitated by our having a new CEO in place, and if the initiative had higher priority for the board chair, who has been preoccupied with matters relating to alliances or merger of the hospital or medical center with other hospitals and health care systems. An alternative slower strategy involves persuading a critical segment of the board and of top management that change is realistic and in their interest. The process could be helped as well by voluntary guidelines set by accreditors or regulators.

The problems in implementing such change are daunting. First, there is overcoming inertia, otherwise known as "there are more important things to do." Second, key members of the powers that be may see the proposed change as criticism aimed at how they have been doing their job, while benefits appear vague relative to the very real costs in obtaining the data and spending scarce board time together to discuss the data. And there may be disagreement as to what board functions are. Third, critical indicators are only as good as they are

Table 11.1.   Medical Center Performance Scorecard, 1998

| Performance Indicator | Record of Performance | | |
	Actual[a]	Targeted[b]	Variance[c]
Financial			
Excess of revenues over expenses	$2.709 million	$1.076	152%
Cash and investments	$7.802 million	$6.758	15%
Number of discharges	17,324	17,348	(0.1%)
Medical loss ratio (HMO)	72.42%	80.85%	10%
Growth and development			
Case mix index	1.32	1.38	(4%)
Number inpatient surgical procedures	3,882	4,373	(11%)
Ambulatory care visits (thousands)	438.7	409.7	7%
Managed care member months (thousands)	456.2	497.2	(8%)
Quality			
Significant patient incidents (hospital)	0	0	
Cesarean section rates	21.6%	20.7%	(4%)
Patients without pressure sores (NH)	96.0%	95+ %	1%
Immunization rate (HMO)	82.0%	87.0%	(5%)
Customer satisfaction			
Inpatients (hospital)	3.32[d]	3.51	(5%)
Outpatients (Health Center)	88.0%	90%	
Employees (hospital and Health Center)	80.0%	95%	
HMO members	97.0%	99%	

Note: HMO = health maintenance organization; NH = nursing home.

[a] Represents actual figures.

[b] Targets chosen based on a variety of sources such as the institution's strategic plan, New York State Department of Health data, or the comparative data base used by a national company carrying out patient surveys.

[c] Percentages are determined by dividing the actual percentage number into the difference between actual and target. For example, the actual medical loss ratio (72.2%) divided by the difference (8.43%) = 10%.

[d] Scale of satisfaction is 1 to 5, with 5 = highly satisfied.

used in board decision making. Getting the data and reflecting on indicator scores does not seem worthy of the costs, unless the board continuously reflects on whether these are the most important indicators and on whether remediable interventions are being made and regularly reported upon either to change performance or further adapt the indicators. I remain convinced that any effective board will regularly review the information that it receives as to whether this is what the board requires to effectively carry out its functions.

NOTES

1. A. R. Kovner, "Governance and Management," in *Health Care Delivery in the United States*, ed. A. R. Kovner and S. Jonas (New York: Springer, 1999).

2. Richard Umbdenstock and W. M. Hageman, "The Five Critical Areas for Effective Governance of Not-for-Profit Hospitals," *Hospital and Health Services Administration* 35, no. 4 (1990): 481–92. And see D. D. Pointer, J. A. Alexander, and H. S. Zuckerman, "The Governance Challenge: Preserving Community Mission with Integrated Health Care Systems," *Frontiers of Health Services Management* 11, no. 3 (spring 1995): 9–10.

3. Ernst & Young, *Shining Light on Your Board's Passage to the Future* (Chicago: Ernst & Young, 1997).

4. J. R. Knickman, "Futures," in *Health Care Delivery in the United States*, ed. Kovner and Jonas.

5. A. R. Kovner, "Health Maintenance Organizations and Managed Care," in *Health Care Delivery in the United States*, ed. Kovner and Jonas.

6. William Bowen, *Inside the Boardroom: Governance by Directors and Trustees* (New York: Wiley, 1994), 18–20. Also see Dennis D. Pointer and Charles M. Ewell, *Really Governing: How Health System and Hospital Boards Can Make More of a Difference* (Albany, N.Y.: Delmar, 1994), 64.

7. Miriam M. Wood, "Introduction: Governance and Leadership in Theory and Practice," in *Nonprofit Boards and Leadership*, ed. Miriam M. Wood (San Francisco: Jossey-Bass, 1996), 1–14.

8. John Carver, *Boards That Make a Difference* (San Francisco: Jossey-Bass, 1990), 16.

9. Shoshonna Sofaer, J. Lammers, and N. Pourat, "What Do We Really Know about the Impact of Board on Nonprofit Hospital Performance," *Journal of Health Administration Education*, 9, no. 4 (fall 1991): 425–42.

10. Bowen, *Inside the Boardroom*, 18–20.

11. Pointer and Ewell, *Really Governing*, 64.

12. D. D. Pointer, J. A. Alexander, and H. S. Zuckerman, "The Governance Challenge: Preserving Community Mission with Integrated Health Care Systems," *Frontiers of Health Services Management* 11, no. 3 (spring 1995): 9–10.

13. John R. Griffith, Vinod K. Sahney, and Ruth A. Mohr, *Reengineering Health Care: Building on CQI* (Ann Arbor, Mich.: Health Administration Press, 1995), 137–38.

14. J. E. Orlikoff and M. K. Totten, "Trustee Workbook, Board Oversight of Quality," *Trustee* 49, no. 4 (April 1996), supplement: 1–4.

15. John R. Griffith, *The Well-Managed Healthcare Organization,* 4th ed. (Chicago: Health Administration Press, 1999), 18.

16. J. E. Orlikoff and M. K. Totten, "Information and the Effective Board," in *The Trustee Guide to Strategic Planning and Information in Health Care* (Chicago: AHA Press, 1998).

17. W. G. MacKaye, "Checking the Dashboard," *In Trust,* summer 1993, 17.

18. MGH Hotline, "MGH Vital Signs," January 24, 1997.

19. R. S. Kaplan and D. P. Norton, "Using the Balanced Scoreboard as a Strategic Management System," *Harvard Business Review,* January–February 1996, 75–85.

12

WHAT HOSPITAL TRUSTEES CAN LEARN FROM ETHICS COMMITTEES

Pragmatism, Ethics, and the Governance of Health Care Organizations

Joseph J. Fins

HYMAN'S LEGACY

In 1963, William A. Hyman, a member of the board of directors of the Jewish Chronic Disease Hospital in Brooklyn, New York, took his institution to court.[1] He had learned that physicians on the hospital's staff had injected live cancer cells into twenty-two chronically ill patients in an experiment designed to assess the immune response. Hyman was concerned that studies were conducted without the consent of the patients and that these experiments could place them at risk. He brought his concerns to his fellow board members but was unable to mobilize support for his position. Instead of finding sympathetic colleagues, he encountered an intransigent institution unwilling to address his allegations of ethical improprieties. He was not allowed to review the medical records of study patients, and instead he encountered what he characterized as a well-orchestrated "whitewash."

Stymied by hospital administration and frustrated by his fellow board members, Hyman sought judicial relief. He filed suit to obtain information about the experiments and their authorization. In a petition to the court, Hyman articulated his responsibility, as a trustee, "to protect the integrity of the hospital." He asserted that

> it is his obligation as a director of said hospital to inquire into such happenings and to ascertain all the facts, and to take adequate steps to protect the patients of the hospital and the good name and reputation of the hospital and of the directors and of the physicians connected with the hospital, and to avoid any possibility of liability on the part of the hospital and of the directors as a result of any injury that may be suffered by any patient as a result of said injections.[2]

Through word and deed, Hyman demonstrated that hospital trustees have the ultimate responsibility for the ethical integrity of the institutions that they serve. His statement to the court articulates the ethical obligations of hospital trusteeship: gathering information necessary for governance; fiduciary protection of patients entrusted to the hospital's care; maintaining the good name of the institution, directors, and staff; and protecting the hospital from liability. These are not only the responsibilities of administrators or clinical staff but above all of the board of trustees—or, in this case, one member of the board, when institutional integrity was at stake.

Hyman v. Jewish Chronic Disease Hospital plays a prominent role in the history of medical ethics; so much so that it is the subject of the opening chapter in Jay Katz's landmark book on research ethics, *Experimentation with Human Beings*. This legacy is significant and is a tribute to the memory of an individual trustee who understood his fiduciary role and associated obligations.

Hyman sounded his alarm sixteen years after the promulgation of the Nuremberg Code,[3] three years before Henry Beecher's exposé of research abuses published in mainstream medical journals[4] and a full nine years before the Tuskegee syphilis study revelations.[5] He addressed a fundamental ethical concern of his era. Responsibly, as a member of his board, he saw a wrong and tried to right it—first within the grievance process, and then through a judicial remedy that history has recognized as important and pivotal. Indeed, his actions point to the centrality of trustees, collectively and individually, to the ethical integrity of a hospital.

His actions led the New York State Court of Appeals to uphold a lower court ruling granting Hyman access to the medical records of the patients who had received the injections. Writing for the court, Chief Judge Desmond ruled "that petitioner, being a director of a hospital corporation, is entitled as a matter of law to an inspection of the records of the hospital to investigate into the facts of alleged illegal and improper experimentation on patients." Desmond further opined that in representing the interests of patients by seeking their records, "He is carrying out his duties as a director—to direct the affairs of the corporation."[6]

Two of the doctors involved in this research were found to have engaged in professional misconduct because they withheld information from subjects and did not obtain informed consent for their studies. Although papers resulting from these studies were published in the medical literature,[7] Dr. Chester M. Southam of the Sloan-Kettering Institute for Cancer Research and Memorial Hospital and Dr. Emanuel E. Mandel, Director of the Department of Medicine at the Jewish Chronic Disease Hospital, were disciplined by the Board of Regents of the University of the State of New York for professional misconduct. The Regents suspended their licenses to practice medicine, stayed their suspensions, and placed both physicians on probation for a year.

In the intervening years since *Hyman v. Jewish Chronic Disease Hospital*, much has changed in research and clinical ethics. Institutional review boards have been established to oversee research ethics, and hospital ethics committees that protect patient rights have become a regular feature of organizational life. But even with these developments, we can continue to learn from the example set by William Hyman about the role of hospital trustees and the obligations of governance.

TRUSTEE STEWARDSHIP TODAY

If the trustee today remains a fiduciary as he was in Hyman's day, the objects of his or her advocacy have changed. Today the challenges are more complex. They transcend the clinical and involve organizational ethics and the ethical integrity of systems of care. Today, the challenges involve macroeconomic questions like stewardship in a complex environment marked by the emergence of managed care, decreased hospital subsides from state and federal governments, and rising costs of technology and increased need for capital. These concerns force the trustee to consider dramatic questions such as hospital closure, hospital conversion to nonprofit foundations, and institutional mergers. Institutional responses to these pressures can have a profound impact on hospitals. They can prompt reorganizations that disrupt patient care and distract staff from their clinical responsibilities. Downsizings and staff reductions can demoralize clinical staff and place patients at risk. Such actions have led California recently to legislate minimum nurse-to-patient ratios to ensure adequate staff.[8] Institutional responses to these economic pressures can eviscerate leading medical programs through the use of outside consultants hired to "slash and burn" academic medical centers.[9]

All these actions have the potential to place patients at risk and to imperil great medical institutions that have been built over decades and centuries. The historic legacy of generations of philanthropic trustees who saw the hospital as "a place of service"—to borrow Rosemary Stevens's phrase[10]—has been placed at risk as we enter the twenty-first century confronted by new economic and policy realities.

In spite of these changes, or perhaps because of them, the central ethical obligations of the trustee have been codified in hospital accreditation standards. The Joint Commission on Accreditation of Healthcare Organizations (JCAHO) has articulated the obligations of hospital trustees. JCAHO's 1998 Accreditation Standards state that working with senior leadership, the governing body or board "has ultimate authority for establishing policy, maintaining quality of care, and for providing for organizational management and planning."[11] Prominent among these responsibilities is the centrality of patients' rights and organizational ethics in institutional life. These themes are not a peripheral issue for accreditation but ones given high visibility in the accreditation standards and during the hospital site visit.

As understood by JCAHO, patients' rights and organizational ethics encompass a far broader area of concern than individual care decisions such as whether a patient is extubated from a ventilator or whether care is futile or not. In today's hospital setting, ethical concerns exist at the micro level of patient care all the way up to questions of organizational ethics and policies. At the level of clinical ethics, this entails providing assistance with the care decisions for individual patients and their families through an ethics consultation service, a bioethics consultant, or an ethics committee. Policy work involves the drafting of policies and procedures and educating staff about patients' rights, privacy, confidentiality, informed consent and informed refusal, decisions near the end of life (e.g., policies to withhold or withdraw life-sustaining therapies), brain death, and organ donation, among others.

More recently, JCAHO has become interested in the issue of organizational ethics and corporate compliance with legal and ethical norms. This level of concern centers on broader organizational dimensions of institutional life, including issues such as the promulgation of practices that are consistent with the institutional mission and core values statement. Specifically, JCAHO expects institutions to have policies and operational mechanisms to address issues such as the integrity of clinical decisions in a cost-conscious environment; conflict resolution; staff conscientious objection; conflict of interest; fair marketing and billing practices; community service; clinical competency; regulation of human subjects research; and compliance with applicable law. Institutional ethics committees, working in tandem with institutional review boards that regulate research, have a major responsibility for ensuring compliance with these clinical and organizational ethics standards.

ETHICS COMMITTEES AND GOVERNANCE

To help fulfill the regulatory expectations laid out by JCAHO and to fulfill the normative mandate of trusteeship, hospital boards need reliable information and assistance in using this information to make governance decisions that invariably involve choices between competing goods. A hospital's ethics committee can assist the board in two ways. First, working through sanctioned channels, the ethics committee can provide the board with information about the clinical context and the provision of care that will be essential for responsible governance decisions. Second, given their expertise in moral reasoning, committee members can provide guidance when directors must make choices between competing goods.

The Centrality of Information

If there was an implicit lesson in the *Hyman v. Jewish Chronic Disease Hospital*, it was that trustees need information to fulfill the mandate of governance. In Hyman's case, he needed access to the charts of patients who were part of Dr. Southam's study. In complex health care settings, modern trustees need information about the fiscal state of the institution as well as the internal care environment where patient care is delivered.

It is self-evident that the quality of information possessed by the board will influence the quality of the decisions they make. Unfortunately, sometimes an information deficit is only identified once missteps have occurred. This is especially true in complex organizations, such as the modern hospital, which develop tiers of management that are progressively distanced from the clinical enterprise.

Both directors and senior administrators are increasingly distracted from clinical operations by the threat of outside competition and the need to negotiate alliances and mergers with other institutions. The focus is directed outward at the marketplace toward managed care reimbursements, and political exigencies such as the impact of the Balanced Budget Amendment—all important variables that will determine the survivability and future of the institution. But this orientation has its costs. It can distract trustees from paying attention to the intramural care environment and the experiences of patients, families, and those providing care.

This distancing from the clinical realm is further complicated by the fact that trustees neither routinely live in the communities served by the hospital nor receive care there. Boards that were once local enterprises and representative of neighborhood communities are now frequently constituted to satisfy the political exigencies of strategic alliances between merged or affiliated institutions.

Focused upon externalities, boards can become prone to make errors in judgment that will affect the clinical enterprise. To counter this possibility, rapidly growing institutions need to enhance mechanisms to inform the board about clinical operations. The ethics committee structure can provide an additional perspective on institutional life and supplement the information supplied to the board, by more traditional sources such as senior management, the medical board, and quality assurance committees.

Ethics committees can provide this perspective because of their composition and the kind of work they do within institutions. Although composition varies across institutions, these committees are typically comprised of physicians, nurses, social workers, chaplains, and administrators, as well as hospital counsel and community members. They have a broad range of responsibilities including ethics case consultation, staff, and the drafting of policies and procedures that pertain to patients' rights and organizational ethics.

Furthermore, these committees are often a vertical slice through the institution, with both senior and junior staff represented. Because ethics committee work is premised upon the notion that all its members are moral agents entitled to voice an opinion about ethically contentious issues, both senior and junior members are able to voice their views. For this reason, the normal hierarchies that exist in institutional life, though not eliminated, are reduced in the setting of the ethics committee, thus making discourse more honest and forthright. This candor can often reveal problems that may only be apparent to a junior staff person who directly provides care or works a night shift.

Operationally the committee is not departmentally based but charged with an institution-wide mandate. Therefore, ethics committees command a hospital-wide perspective that allows them to identify systems problems that may involve more than one department. Such an interdepartmental perspective can be of assistance to boards that often fall victim to a fragmented view of organizational life. In his book, *Boards That Make a Difference*, Carver warns against the fragmentation that can occur when: "a board faces a sequence of disconnected and unmanageably voluminous vertical slices of the whole instead of a holistic, manageable fabric of horizontally connected policies. We all profess that boards should view the big picture. Yet what most boards confront in meeting after meeting are pieces that are too specific."[12]

Because the work of ethics committees tends to integrate—rather than fragment—organizational life, knowledge of their work can serve as a helpful "structural conduit" between the clinical arena and the board.[13]

Envisioning a Structural Conduit between the Ethics Committee and the Board

Having argued that promoting periodic ethics committee interaction with the board can improve their deliberative process as fiduciaries, it is important to note that these exchanges are useful only if senior leadership agrees that the board should interact with the ethics committee. The hospital administration needs to sanction these exchanges and make arrangements that are appropriate given the prevailing institutional culture.

This dialogue could be accomplished in a number of ways, including trustee membership on the ethics committee, periodic reports of the ethics committee to the quality-assurance subcommittee to the board, or presentations and/or consultations with the full board. Each of these alternatives has its merits and limitations.

Trustee membership on the ethics committee may be an ideal strategy to promote dialogue between the committee and the board. Trustees who serve on the committee will gain a firsthand appreciation of the committee's work and the resources that could be made available to the board. Furthermore, trustee committee members can help promote a level of trust that would be necessary for the full board to feel comfortable consulting with the committee over sensitive matters. Conversely, the ethics committee may gain greater insight into the work of the board and the institution's goals and mission. It may also be enriched by having a distinguished community member partake in its deliberations.

Trustee membership on the board, however, must be arranged with great care so as to avoid the appearance that staff is attempting to circumvent normal channels of communication through administration. Trustee membership must be vetted and approved by senior administration. In addition, the board will need to determine whether trustee membership on the ethics committee makes the best use of the limited time and resource of its members.

Periodic ethics committee reports to the board are less helpful than trustee membership on the committee. No reporting mechanism can replace trustee representation on the committee. Nonetheless, there are clear advantages to regular reports to the board. Periodic reporting helps to formalize and expand the relationship beyond the individual board member who serves on the committee. In the absence of actual trustee membership, these reports can make the full board aware of committee activities and areas of inquiry.

In addition to these activities, personal appearances by the ethics committee chair before the board can be extremely useful. This can build relationships and foster trust necessary for more involved consultation. It is important to appreciate that consultations over difficult issues are not likely to occur de novo without a history of productive interactions between the board and the ethics committee. It is important to build these relationships before the need for more intensive ethics committee–board dialogue arises.

GUIDANCE IN MORAL REASONING: CLINICAL PRAGMATISM

In most institutions, senior management is adept at providing information about the financial state of the institution. Board members who generally come from the business community are skilled at interpreting this information. Hospital boards are less adept, however, at making ethical judgments, and they often fail to appreciate that their decisions have an ethical dimension.

This problem is not unique to hospital boards but rather a feature of the unique challenge of serving on a not-for-profit board. William G. Bowen, in his book *Inside the Boardroom*, quotes a senior administrator at a prominent museum who observes that service on a not-for-profit board presents challenges to business trustees who are being asked to play roles that "raise unfamiliar types of normative questions." Bowen comments:

> Informed decisions in such situations require rather sophisticated understanding of the implications of not spending money, as well as spending it, and a willingness to make hard intergenerational choices: What will be the long-term effects of either decision on the quality of the institution. . . . Corporations also make present-versus-future choices all the time, but at least they have quantitative methodologies to guide them in framing the issues and projecting rates of return.[14]

Ethics committees, which are accustomed to working with "normative questions," can be a resource in moral reasoning for the board by providing a methodology to consider the ethical implications of governance decisions. This is especially important when the board must consider issues where the choices are neither clear, right or wrong, but rather where there is a need to balance several goods, values, and interests. In such cases, ethical governance is not found in a particular outcome but rather in the quality of the process of deliberations. The ethics structure in the hospital can assist in this deliberative process and help promote a process of systematic and thoughtful inquiry.

Clinical pragmatism—a method of moral problem solving that my colleagues and I have developed for addressing ethical issues in practice[15]—can serve as a model for "pragmatic inquiry" in board deliberations. This method can be helpful to boards in their governance process. Clinical pragmatism should not be confused with the vernacular usage of pragmatism, which connotes expediency. Instead, clinical pragmatism is a structured method of moral problem solving in the American pragmatic tradition, most significantly drawing upon the philosophical legacy of John Dewey (1859–1952).[16] Dewey was a democratic theorist, pragmatist, and education reformer who stressed the interdependence of theory and practice.[17]

Dewey's reliance upon inductive reasoning and his quest to integrate theory and practice in a way that would have a bearing on real life situations makes his work an ideal foundation for ethical problem solving in the clinical setting or in not-for-profit governance. Furthermore, Dewey's concern about the centrality of consensus in normative deliberations is especially relevant to boards that need to govern with a unified voice to provide unequivocal guidance for senior management and staff.

Like Dewey's pragmatism, clinical pragmatism is not ethical theory founded upon fixed absolute truths, but is instead a process of inquiry that admits fallibility and contingency—characteristics particularly well suited to governance decisions made for complex health care organizations. Clinical pragmatism views ethical principles as hypotheses that need to be validated by their consequences for practice. When only a single ethical principle is in play, it can guide conduct. But in more complex deliberations when two or more principles are at odds, clinical pragmatism focuses on the promotion of what Dewey called "inquiry."

Inquiry begins with the recognition of a problematic situation that calls for further examination. A morally problematic situation is one that needs deeper consideration because ethical tensions are present but as yet unexplored. The goal is to make implicit assumptions, goals, and conflicts explicit so as to allow everyone involved to come to a clear recognition of a problem and to engage in a thorough analysis of it. This will lead to a better outcome. Although problematic situations are evident in retrospect, they are not self-evident moving forward.

The recognition of a potentially problematic situation is dependent upon an adequate stream of information to the board so that it can preemptively address potentially difficult situations. My earlier recommendation to use the ethics committee as a structural conduit for information for the board was to assist the board in its important function of identifying problematic situations in a timely manner so that staff and board resources can be directed to their analysis.

This analysis is a series of related steps that can occur in sequence (or simultaneously) through a contextually situated analysis. In this process, the objective is to consider the range of facts necessary to reach a judgment about a reasonable course of action. Before any decision is made, pragmatic inquiry requires that boards review pertinent facts; identify stakeholders and hear their positions; reflect on institutional values; consider contextual organizational factors; and place these deliberations within any larger societal issues.

Once boards have collected this comprehensive array of information, they can begin to consider the range of reasonable moral considerations that might bear upon the development of a workable consensus to resolve the moral problem. In clinical practice, this process is the formulation of an ethics differential diagnosis. Just as physicians create a differential diagnosis that centers on complaints, signs, symptoms, physical findings, and laboratory tests, so too the application of clinical pragmatism to governance issues centers upon the range of reasonable decisions a board can make.

The analog to differential diagnosis in governance is nicely illustrated by the work of board subcommittees charged by the full board with an in-depth examination of a particular problem and to report back with a number of alternatives. In his volume on board process and function, Carver implicitly endorses the value of the differential diagnosis when discussing the optimal way boards can utilize the work of subcommittees charged with addressing specific issues for later consideration by the full board. He observes that: "If a board is to deliberate and adopt a policy position, it will do a better job if several options are available. Having only one option is a flaw inherent in the recommendation practice. The availability of several alternatives, however, will not necessarily lead to an intelligent choice unless the board is aware of the implications of each option. In other words, the board needs to know the choices and the consequences of these choices. Only then can it ponder, debate, and vote intelligently."[18]

Boards should collect the facts and view future governance decisions as hypotheticals that need to be validated in practice and through the reaching of a consensus. This inductive process will not guarantee a "right" decision. But the pragmatic deliberative process outlined here will increase the probability that a reasonable outcome will occur and that interests of relevant stakeholders will be identified and given voice.

Once the options have been presented to the board, it is the task of board members to come to a decision about governance. It is in this stage of deliberations that Dewey's linking of an empirical method with the deliberative process that leads to a workable consensus is so helpful for governance. Dewey explained the instrumentality of his method in *Experience and Nature*:

> The adoption of an empirical method is no guarantee that all the things relevant to any particular conclusion will actually be found, or that when found they will be correctly shown and communicated. But empirical method points out when and where and how things of a designated description have been arrived at. It places before others a map of the road that has been traveled; they may accordingly, if they will, re-travel the road to inspect the landscape for themselves. Thus the findings of one may be rectified and extended by the findings of others, with as much assurance as is humanly possible of confirmation, extension and rectification. The adoption of empirical method thus procures for philosophic reflection something of that cooperative tendency toward consensus which marks inquiry in the natural sciences. The scientific investigator convinces others not by the plausibility of his definitions and the cogency of his dialectic, but by placing before them the specified course of searchings, doings, and arrivals, in consequence of which certain things have been found. His appeal is for others to traverse a similar course, so as to see how what they find corresponds with his report.[19]

Pragmatic inquiry is especially well suited to board deliberations because of the importance of reaching consensus on governance issues. A board that is not united in its strategic decisions is one that sends out mixed signals. If we imagine a hospital board that reaches a decision by a 20-to-15 vote, we can envision a health care organization that will shortly find itself in crisis. This certainly was the case in *Hyman v. Chronic Jewish Disease Hospital* when a lone board member took the hospital to court. More generally, board discord is disruptive to organizational life. Staff and other interested observers of the board vote will try to ferret out which board faction or alliance was ascendant, and which was in decline and what these votes mean for present and future administrations. Such speculations breed a climate of uncertainty and promote discord.

While pragmatic inquiry cannot always promote board harmony, it can minimize discord by making explicit the facts, arguments, and lines of inquiry that led board members to reach a judgment one way or another. By making this process explicit, boards can minimize disagreements that might center on misconstruals or mistaken interpretations. Pragmatic inquiry can also help boards recognize that the lack of consensus or outright discord may herald a problematic situation that requires additional inquiry and a postponement of a vote. A hospital board employing pragmatic deliberations might better appreciate the consequences of a 20-to-15 vote and decide unanimously to table the issue and engage in more fact gathering or debate.

Once a board reaches a consensus, pragmatic inquiry can provide a helpful framework for assessing an intervention. Because pragmatism appreciates that all judgments are contingent, they value periodic review and reassessment of whether their theoretical hypotheses are confirmed by practical results. A board committed to pragmatic inquiry will engage in periodic review and focus on outcome assessments to see whether governance decisions led to fruitful programs for the institution. If this approach is stated at the outset of a new initiative, it will be less difficult to engage in assessment retrospectively.

PRAGMATISM AND GOVERNANCE: A CASE VIGNETTE

To further describe this method, let me delineate this process of inquiry through the consideration of a problem that a hospital board may be asked to address. Although a fictional case vignette cannot do justice to an actual governance decision, this exercise can illustrate the instrumental value of a structured process of inquiry.

Consider the following hypothetical situation.[20] Two hospitals have recently merged in the face of challenging market forces in the hope that a unified institution—with a greater percentage of market share—will be better poised to negotiate favorable contracts with managed care companies. With the merger has come some level of redundancy in clinical services. The hospital chief executive officer, desiring to stem a budget deficit, asks the board to consider consolidating the psychiatric services at the two hospitals and locating them at a single site.

Problematic Situation

At the outset, it is important to recognize that this consolidation, prompted by market pressures, is indeed an ethically problematic situation.[21] Although some board members might view the consolidation of psychiatric services as a welcome financial benefit of having a merged institution, a fiscal analysis alone is inadequate. When considering this governance decision more comprehensively, the board would need to make explicit the implicit assumptions that led the organization to promote this consolidation. A helpful first question might be: Why consolidate psychiatry instead of pediatrics or a cardiac surgery program?

At the outset, it would be important to know whether the decision was prompted by biases toward the mentally ill or an undervaluing of the psychiatric enterprise as compared with other fields in medicine. Even more fundamentally, the board would need to question the premise that the services offered by the two psychiatric units were indeed overlapping and redundant. More generic to the psychology of mergers, a board engaged in assessing this sort of consolidation would also want to know whether personality issues played into this decision and whether the site for the consolidated service was already chosen, and if so why. Did power dynamics stemming from the merger lead to this decision?

The board would also need to consider what would be lost if the two programs consolidated. While the merger might lead to some savings—an assumption that would need to be demonstrated—what would be the programmatic disadvantages of a single psychiatric service? Would a consolidation of the two services be consistent with the institution's mission statement to "provide outstanding medical care, promote biomedical research, and foster medical education"? Seen in this light, a board would need to ask whether the consolidation would decrease the institution's ability to serve the mentally ill and whether it would adversely effect the hospital's research and postgraduate training programs in psychiatry.

Pertinent Facts

With these issues in mind, a board subcommittee could begin its process of inquiry and ensure that management's recommendation to consolidate the two services was founded upon an adequate assessment of medical, public health, and scientific data. Given the hypothetical nature of this example, I can only suggest some of the questions that might emerge when considering this consolidation. For example, the board subcommittee would want to be assured that management had assessed the impact of the consolidation upon the ability to serve the mentally ill and that patients currently treated at one site would have access to the other. How would this decision influence access or continuity of care? Assuming that patients at one site could travel to the other, are all services at one campus available at the other? Are there any special research initiatives at the closing site that should be retained or relocated?

Stakeholders and Spokespersons

Although it is not the purview of the board to speak with all the stakeholders affected by such an initiative, it is their role to be sure that management adequately engaged such individuals. At the clinical level, the board would want to be sure that management had adequately consulted with the chiefs of the two psychiatric services and their key staff to ascertain their views.[22] In addition, the board subcommittee would want to hear of the reactions of patients, their families, and advocacy groups, such as the local chapter of the National Alliance for the Mentally Ill. Finally, the board would want to be informed by the hospital's office of sponsored and philanthropic programs about the impact of the proposed consolidation on fund raising and grant support and for the academic initiatives of the two services.[23]

Contextual Factors

When considering the organizational implications of the consolidation of the psychiatric services, a board subcommittee should seek to ensure that the cost–benefit analysis provided by management adequately modeled all the gains and liabilities imposed by this decision.[24] For example, management would need to demonstrate how the closure of one psychiatric service would influence the institution's global budget. While a closure might save money when seen from the narrow vantage point of psychiatry, would a closure at one site decrease revenue streams from other services or increase the cost of providing psychiatric care in nonpsychiatric departments? Furthermore, a board would need to assure itself that consolidation would not adversely influence the institution's ability to seek a managed care contract, given the presence of a single site for the provision of care.[25] Finally, for a board to approve such a decision, it would need to be confident that any monies saved in the closure of a psychiatric service would be put to better use elsewhere in the system. If a more beneficial use for those dollars could not be demonstrated, a board would be ill advised to support such a drastic measure.

Institutional Values

Given the mission statement's commitment to serving the needs of patients, medical education, and research, the board should reflect on how this decision fits with institutional values and the hospital's historic role and responsibilities.[26] More speculatively, governance would need to consider how their decision might influence the quest for meaning in institutional life and the aspirations and hopes of those associated with the institution.[27] At a more practical level, it would need to assess how a consolidation of services might affect the use of any restricted philanthropic funds given to support the psychiatric service.

Extramural and Societal Issues

Because decisions like this one are often reflective of broader social currents, the board would need to be aware of whether any external biases or fears related to mental illness were influencing administration's recommendation for consolidation.[28] In this context, it would be reasonable to ask why and how psychiatry was chosen for downsizing. In addition, a prudent board would look beyond its own institutional experience and see how similar consolidations had fared in other settings.[29]

An Organizational Differential Diagnosis and Consensus

Once a board subcommittee has studied this issue and worked with administration, it is time for a report to the full board to reach a consensus. To facilitate this process, the subcommittee could outline a number of reasonable recommendations. Offering the board a number of alternative solutions to the problem will help promote inquiry and lead to a better decision-making process to the institution. In this hypothetical, a board subcommittee might recommend three alternatives: (1) outright closure of one psychiatric service; (2) keeping both sites open and functioning; (3) keep both sites operational but shift the bulk of programmatic activities to a single location.

Whatever the board subcommittee recommends, it is important that it outline its thinking in support of its recommendations so that fellow board members can follow the logic of the smaller working group. This will help ensure that the full board is working with the same data and operating assumptions. This will also promote consensus and lead to unified governance.

Implementation, Evaluation, and Periodic Review

Once the board reaches a decision with respect to the consolidation of the psychiatric services, pragmatic inquiry can be helpful in assessing the results and modifying the course of action. Because outcomes may involve intangibles that may be more difficult to quantify than the bottom line, boards engaged in this pragmatic process of inquiry would seek to outline outcome measures prospectively that could be used to gauge programmatic success or failure. Such indicators might include patient volumes on the consolidated psychiatric services, the number of faculty members in the departments of psychiatry, and the volume of research grants they secured. Outcomes might also assess more qualitative outcomes such as patient satisfaction and perceived ease of access to psychiatric care. By organizing these empirical observations, senior management can provide governance with information that will help to productively reconstruct practice.

CONCLUSION

The challenges facing trustees are profound and historic. Their choices will shape the health care system that our children will inherit. Given this responsibility, we must ensure that trustees are well informed and well equipped for their deliberations. They need accurate information about the care environment and guidance in a deliberative process that will involve ethical choices. Although the deliberations of trustees will be grounded in economics, their choices will be fundamentally ethical ones that involve competing goods. By involving the institutional ethics committee in this process of inquiry and deliberation, health care organizations will be better able to find meaning in institutional life and transform the mission statement from a series of platitudes to a strategic vision that will help maintain institutional integrity during a time of unparalleled change.

NOTES

1. J. Katz, *Experimentation with Human Beings* (New York: Russell Sage Foundation. 1972), 7–65.

2. Katz, *Experimentation*, 12.

3. *Trials of War Criminals before the Nuremburg Military Tribunals under Control Council Law No. 10*, vol. 2 (Washington, D.C.: U.S. Government Printing Office, 1949).

4. Henry K. Beecher, "Ethics and Clinical Research," *New England Journal of Medicine* 274 (1966): 1354–60.

5. J. H. Jones, *Bad Blood*, 2d ed. (New York: Free Press, 1983).

6. Katz, *Experimentation*, 44–45.

7. A. G. Levin, D. B. Custodio, E. E. Mandel, and C. M. Southam, "Rejection of Cancer Homotransplants by Patients with Debilitating Non-Neoplastic Diseases," *Annals of the New York Academy of Science* 120 (1964): 410–23.

8. California Nurses Association Press Release. Governor signs safe hospital staffing law; www.californianurses.org/cna/press/101099.html, October 10, 1999.

9. M. Freudheim, "Bitter Pill for Ailing Hospitals," *New York Times*. October 31, 1999, section 3, p. 1.

10. R. Stevens, *In Sickness and in Wealth* (New York: Basic Books. 1989), 38.

11. Joint Commission on Accreditation of Healthcare Organizations, *1998 Hospital Accreditation Standards* (Oakbrook Terrace, Ill.: Joint Commission on Accreditation of Healthcare Organizations. 1998), 215–19.

12. J. Carver, *Boards That Make a Difference: A New Design for Leadership in Nonprofit and Public Organizations*, 2nd ed. (San Francisco: Jossey-Bass. 1997), 47.

13. I am indebted to Pat Levinson for this phrase.

14. William G. Bowen, *Inside the Boardroom* (New York: John Wiley & Sons, 1994), 138–39.

15. J. J. Fins and M. D. Bacchetta, "Framing the Physician-Assisted Suicide and Voluntary Active Euthanasia Debate: The Role of Deontology, Consequentialism, and Clinical Pragmatism," *Journal of the American Geriatrics Society* 43, no. 5 (1995): 563–68. J. J. Fins, "From Indifference to Goodness," *Journal of Religion and Health* 35, no. 3 (1996): 245–54. J. J. Fins, M. D. Bacchetta, and F. G. Miller, "Clinical Pragmatism: A Method of Moral Problem Solving," *Kennedy Institute of Ethics Journal* 7, no. 2 (1997): 129–45. F. G. Miller, J. C. Fletcher, and J. J. Fins, "Clinical Pragmatism: A Case Method of Moral Problem Solving," *Introduction to Clinical Ethics*, 2d edition, ed. J. C. Fletcher, P. A. Lombardo, M. F. Marshal, and F. G. Miller (Frederick, Md.: University Publishing Group. 1997). J. J. Fins, "Approximation and Negotiation: Clinical Pragmatism and Difference," *Cambridge Quarterly of Healthcare Ethics* 7, no. 1 (1998): 68–76. J. J. Fins, F. G. Miller, and M. D. Bacchetta, "Clinical Pragmatism: Bridging Theory and Practice," *Kennedy Institute of Ethics Journal* 8, no. 1(1998): 39–44. J. J. Fins and F. G. Miller, "Clinical Pragmatism, Ethics Consultation and the Elderly," *Clinics in Geriatrics*, no. 16 (2000): 71–81.

16. S. Hook, *John Dewey: An Intellectual Portrait* (Amherst, N.Y.: Prometheus Books, 1995). F. G. Miller, J. J. Fins, and M. D. Bacchetta, "Clinical Pragmatism: John Dewey and Clinical Ethics," *Journal of Contemporary Health Law and Policy* 13, no. 27 (1996): 27–51.

17. J. J. Fins, "Klinischer Pragmatismus und Ethik-Konsultation" (Clinical Pragmatism and Ethics Case Consultation), *Das Parlament*, June 4, 1999, 18. John Dewey, "The Logic of Judgments of Practice," *The Essential Dewey: Ethics, Logic, Psychology*, ed. L. A. Hickman and T. M. Alexander (Bloomington: Indiana University Press, 1998), vol. 2, 236–71.

18. J. Carver, *Boards*, 150–51.

19. J. Dewey, *Experience & Nature* (Chicago: Open Court, 1997), 28.

20. This is a hypothetical vignette and does not reflect deliberations or discussions of any institution with which I am affiliated.

21. P. J. Boyle and D. Callahan, "Managed Care in Mental Health: The Ethical Issues," *Health Affairs* 14, no. 3 (1995): 7–22.

22. J. B. Sardis, "Pills, Policies, and Patients," *Health Affairs* 18, no. 5 (1999): 156–62.

23. H. S. Moffic, K. Drieg, and H. Prosen, "Managed Care and Academic Psychiatry," *Journal of Mental Health Administration* 20, no. 2 (1993): 172–77.

24. M. D. Bacchetta and J. J. Fins, "The Economics of Clinical Ethics Programs: A Quantitative Justification," *Cambridge Quarterly of Healthcare Ethics* 6, no. 4 (1997): 451–60.

25. Consider costs carefully before accepting risk for the severely mentally ill. *Capitation Rates Data* 3, no. 8 (1998): 95–96.

26. J. E. Sabin, "Caring about Patients and Caring about Money: The APA Code of Ethics Meets Managed Care," *Behavioral Science Law* 12, no. 4 (1994): 317–30.

27. M. L. Pava, *The Search for Meaning in Organizations: Seven Practical Questions for Ethical Managers* (Westport, Conn.: Quorum Books. 1999).

28. B. G. Link, J. C. Phelan, M. Bresnahan, A. Stueve, and B. A. Pescolido, "Public Conceptions of Mental Illness: Labels, Causes, Dangerousness, and Social Distance," *American Journal of Public Health* 90, no. 9 (1999): 1328–33.

29. R. K. Schreter, "Reorganizing Departments of Psychiatry, Hospitals, and Medical Centers for the 21st Century," *Psychiatric Services* 49, no. 11 (1998): 1429–33.

13

PATIENT SAFETY AND THE ROLE OF HOSPITAL BOARDS

Virginia A. Sharpe

B efore 1999, hospital trustees' attention to error seems to have been directed principally to discrepancies or irregularities in billing either by the institution or its vendors. Since the November 1999 release of the Institute of Medicine (IOM) report *To Err Is Human: Building a Safer Health System*, however, concerns about error have assumed a broader scope.[1] Now, questions regarding medical rather then billing error have moved to the forefront of public and institutional consciousness. As the IOM report reveals, anywhere from 44,000 to 98,000 people die every year as a result of preventable errors in the hospital setting. Using the smaller estimate, deaths from preventable medical mistakes rank above the mortality associated with car accidents, breast cancer, or AIDS and are estimated to result in an overall cost of between $17 billion and $29 billion.[2]

Among other things, the IOM recommends that "health care organizations and professionals affiliated with them should make continually improved patient safety a declared and serious aim by establishing patient safety programs with a defined executive responsibility" (Recommendation 8.1).[3] Specifying this recommendation, the IOM explicitly states that "Chief Executive Officers and Boards of Trustees must make a serious and ongoing commitment to creating safe systems of care."[4]

In this chapter, I discuss medical error, the IOM report, and the role that hospital trustees can play in creating a culture of safety in their institutions. I begin with a brief look at the history of the hospital trustee's role with regard to quality. I then discuss boards' contemporary external and internal motivations for quality and patient safety, and I conclude by describing specific actions that boards can take in this role.

HOSPITAL TRUSTEES AND HEALTH CARE QUALITY

As James Orlikoff and Mary Totten have observed, many trustees are uncomfortable with the notion that they bear responsibility for the quality of care within their institutions.[5] Much of this discomfort stems from the fact that since the advent of the modern hospital in the early twentieth century, the quality of hospital care has largely been regarded as a function of the competence and integrity of physicians. This conception of quality has resulted from a combination of practical, political, and financial factors.

In the eighteenth and early nineteenth centuries, decision making in hospitals was the province of the board and was based principally on moral and financial rather than medical considerations.[6] The progress of scientific medicine in the nineteenth and twentieth centuries for the first time distinguished physicians by their expert and often esoteric knowledge. As physicians began to offer an array of hospital-based services, including surgery and later X-ray and laboratory facilities, it seemed impractical and ill-advised to leave clinical decisions to those who were untrained in the clinic. The development and successful use of anesthesia and aseptic techniques drew an unprecedented number of patients to the hospital for surgery that had been rejected as too risky. Increasingly, an institutional affiliation with a surgeon could bring the hospital new admissions and increased revenue.

As doctors gained intellectual primacy in the hospital, they lobbied for increased authority over hospital management and governance. As Charles Rosenberg points out, physicians believed that "clinical and scientific skills were ultimately more central, both to the treatment of individual patients and the making of hospital policy," and they bridled at the experience of their work being overseen by lay trustees.[7] By the early twentieth century, scientific medicine's assumed efficacy and the hospital's dependence on physicians' ability to draw paying patients meant that lay authorities increasingly deferred to physicians and to medical values to assess the quality of medical work.

In the first quarter of the twentieth century, when hospital standards were being developed, emphasis was placed on norms of institutional structure such as staff organization, medical record keeping, and the existence of committees for medical privileges, tissue review, and diagnostic and therapeutic facilities.[8] One rationale for this emphasis was a belief that hospital quality would flow from a hospital's compliance with structural standards. Another rationale conformed to the politics of physician control. Board and executive oversight of quality would be largely concerned with institutional structure; two other dimensions of quality, process and outcome, would largely be left to physicians.[9]

In many ways, today's not-for-profit hospital boards reflect this historical legacy. Beyond retrospective review of quality problems, and review and approval of applications for physician privileges, many boards continue to believe that ensuring the quality of care is the job of the clinical staff.[10] There are a number of important reasons to reject this thinking. These include the board's legal liability; its strategic interests in the competitiveness of its hospital; its interest in its hospital's accreditation; and its moral obligation to prevent patient harm. Let me briefly discuss the first three—what might be understood as external motivations for the board's attention to quality.

EXTERNAL MOTIVATIONS FOR QUALITY

External motivations for quality reflect an institution's accountability to an oversight body. Internal motivations, by contrast, are based on accountability for moral norms that define the practice of patient care. Concerns about legal liability, competitiveness, and accreditation are external motivations.

Legal Liability

The case law has a number of precedents establishing a hospital's direct duty to care for patients. The first case of record is *Darling v. Charleston Community Memorial Hospital*,[11] decided in 1965. In this case, the plaintiff, Dorrence Darling, broke his leg in a college football game and was taken to Charleston Community Memorial Hospital emergency room, where the emergency physician applied traction and put the leg in a plaster cast. Shortly after his leg was placed in the cast, Darling began to experience pain, and his toes protruding from the cast became swollen and discolored. The same emergency doctor removed the cast three days later and cut the patient's leg on both sides. At the time, the nurses noted seepage from the leg and a foul odor. Despite this, the hospital failed to investigate the doctor's work or to request a consultation.

Eleven days later, the plaintiff was transferred to another hospital under the care of an orthopedist and was found to have significant dead tissue on the leg resulting from a lack of circulation and hemorrhaging in the cast. Darling's leg was ultimately amputated below the knee. As the Supreme Court of Illinois observed in this case, "the conception that the hospital does not undertake to act through its doctors and nurses but undertakes instead simply to procure them to act upon their own responsibility, no longer reflects the fact. Present day hospitals, as their manner of operation plainly demonstrates, do far more than furnish facilities for treatment."[12]

In this case, the court held that hospitals and their governing bodies can be held liable for injury resulting from negligent supervision of medical staff members. Subsequent rulings have augmented this precedent through the doctrine of "corporate negligence," establishing that "a hospital has a direct and independent responsibility to its patients; over and above that of the physicians and surgeons participating therein."[13] In recognizing the complexity of modern hospitals and medical centers and the extent to which care is provided through a dynamic system that is greater than the sum of its parts,[14] the courts have recognized the legal liability of the hospital itself and its board regarding the quality of care.

Hospital Competitiveness and Accreditation

The drive to contain health care costs in the United States during the past three decades and the subsequent rise of managed care have together placed unprecedented burdens on hospitals. A sizable percentage of care has shifted from the inpatient to the outpatient setting; hospital reimbursement by private and government insurers has been reduced, thus limiting cross-subsidies for medical education and nonpaying hospital patients. At the same time, charitable giving to not-for-profit hospitals is one of the weakest sectors of American philanthropy.[15] These factors have made it necessary for hospital boards to consider a host of new and challenging financial strategies to keep their institution viable.

Alongside increased fiscal accountability, health care institutions are increasingly called to account for the quality of care they provide. In 1987, the Joint Commission on Accreditation of Healthcare Organizations (JCAHO) instituted a new philosophy of performance measurement designed to move beyond the inferential evaluation of quality through an institution's compliance with structural standards. For the first time in its history, JCAHO endorsed the evaluation of health care quality on the basis of data regarding actual patient outcomes and the processes of hospital work. Behind this new philosophy was the view that quality could be directly measured.[16]

This view has also become a fundamental basis for the evaluation of the quality of managed care plans. The National Commission for Quality Assessment, founded as an independent organization in 1990, uses specific measures (the health plan employer data and information set) as a basis for the comparison of health plan performance. The endorsement of outcomes research as a basis for quality and performance assessment is also reflected in the evolution of the once flagging Agency for Health Care Policy and Research into the robust Agency for Health Care Research and Quality (AHRQ) in 1999. The

IOM's recommendation of a $100 million Center for Patient Safety to, among other things, "set national goals for patient safety" is to be housed within the AHRQ.[17]

As the IOM report makes clear, patient safety is now, and will continue to be, regarded as a critical indicator of health care quality, with the reduction of preventable medical error as a key component. The specific role that patient safety and medical error reduction will play in accreditation and the competitiveness of health care institutions is forecast in the IOM report Recommendation 7.1:

> Performance standards and expectations for health care organizations should focus greater attention on patient safety.
>
> Regulators and accreditors should require health care organizations to implement meaningful patient safety programs with defined executive responsibility.
>
> Public and private purchasers should provide incentives to health care organizations to demonstrate continuous improvement in patient safety.

Several bills have been introduced in Congress proposing legislation to implement the IOM recommendations. Strong bipartisan support and immediate endorsement by President Bill Clinton of the IOM report in 1999 indicate the high level of political support for the institution of external incentives for patient safety. As Kenneth Kizer, president and chief executive officer (CEO) of the National Forum for Health Care Quality and former head of the Veterans Administration has observed, through their leadership, hospital boards and CEOs will play a central role in creating a culture of safety. In the boardroom, says Kiser, "there should be the same level of scrutiny and detail for quality and patient safety as for financials. At every meeting, the board should demand to see the numbers. As far as long-term viability of institutions, [looking at quality] will be critical, based on what's coming down the pike from the government—reporting and safety performance measures. The landscape will change very quickly. Quality will be the Holy Grail of the 21st Century."[18]

In addition to the pragmatic motivations of compliance, accreditation, competitiveness, and fear of legal liability, there are fundamental ethical reasons for boards to take up the cause of patient safety. These ethical reasons can be called "internal" rather then "external" motivations. They reflect the hospital's mission of service to ill people.

Ethical Obligations: Internal Motivations for Quality and Patient Safety

Since the Hippocratic writings of the fourth century B.C., it has been commonly accepted that the healing enterprise is guided by the ethical imperative "to help, or at least to do no harm."[19] Like the conventional wisdom about quality, the conventional wisdom about this basic obligation is that it applies exclusively to clinicians, that is, to physicians and nurses who have direct responsibility for patient care. I have argued elsewhere that this obligation and others that define the fiduciary role of the health care provider to patients should extend beyond doctors and nurses to hospital and health plan administrators, executives, and board members who have an indirect, though significant, influence on patient care.[20] Evidence to support the fiduciary obligation of nonclinical health care providers to patients comes from research on the etiology of harmful medical error.

Since the early 1990s, research on the causes of mistakes in hospitals has revealed that the vast majority of errors are systemic; that is, they stem not from the poor or incompetent performance of individuals but from flaws in the design and function of systems.[21] Look-alike drug labeling or sound-alike drug names may lead to drug errors; an intensive care unit design that does not include convenient hand-washing stations may contribute to the spread of infection; inadequate staffing schedules may lead to sleep deprivation and increase the likelihood of errors of judgment; and a hospital that does not adequately train staff members to use new technologies creates the circumstances under which error will thrive.[22]

All of these examples and the research that supports them underscore one of the basic insights of systems thinking, namely, that "systems function as a whole, so they have properties above and beyond the properties of the parts that comprise them. These are known as emergent properties."[23] On the basis of his work in health care, Lucian Leape, one of the pioneers of patient safety, and his colleagues define "system" as "an interdependent group of items, people or processes with a common purpose."[24] Errors and accidents can be understood as emergent properties of the dynamically complex system of hospital care.

It might seem odd that we have come to this point in a discussion of ethical obligations and patient safety. To define error as "an emergent property of a system" seems by all accounts to overlook the role of human agency and responsibility in error. This seems especially perverse when we think about the ways in which patients are harmed by error in the hospital setting. To clarify this seeming paradox, it is necessary to distinguish between responsibility in the retrospective sense, that is, blame; and responsibility in the prospective sense, that is, responsibility that stems from established goals.

As I noted above, the weight of recent evidence traces most medical error back to system deficiencies. The antidote to error, therefore, is understood to lie in root-cause analysis and system improvement rather than in the surveillance and control of individuals. A systemic problem requires a systemic solution. That having been said, our conventional response to error is look for someone to blame. Both traditional quality assurance and medical malpractice are based on the model of individual agency and responsibility; what Donald Berwick has called the "bad-apple" theory of quality.[25] The theory is that if the poor performers are removed from a system or sufficiently punished, quality will improve. The fear and paranoia generated by this approach to quality have had the effect of silencing discussion of error. This silence, in turn, has obscured potentially preventable problems.[26] Given this, it is widely recognized by leaders in health care quality that "blaming the individual does little to make the system safer"[27] and that a safer system requires changing the culture of blame.

JCAHO has identified at least seven strategies for reducing the risk of harmful medical error in health care institutions: (1) punitive action, (2) retraining/counseling, (3) policy and procedure change, (4) redundant processes, (5) technical system-enhancement, and (6) culture change. Moving down the list, efficacy increases for long-term improvement of patient safety and implementation become more difficult.[28] As those writing on the subject of patient safety and on quality generally have made clear, a system focus within an institution must be spearheaded by institutional leaders.[29] Without that support, the implementation of any change beyond the first three strategies is all but impossible.

A hospital board of trustees thus can play a central role in this cultural change. The board can encourage and support programs that move away from surveillance and blame to analysis that focuses on the root causes of harmful and nonharmful error. The board can make patient safety an integral part of its evaluation of hospital performance. It can support the disclosure and analysis of near-misses—errors that did not cause harm. And it can support institutional change designed to aid in the disclosure of serious adverse events.

It is here that responsibility in the prospective sense shows its relevance. In an argument developed more fully elsewhere, I have described responsibility, in the forward-looking sense, as

> the burden of obligation that accompanies certain roles and offices. When we ask "for what am I responsible?" we are asking about the substantive moral commitments that pertain to the specific practices in which we are engaged; the goals that define the practices and the proper means of attaining them. Responsibility is forward-looking in this sense because it involves prospective reasoning about what I should do and why I should do it rather than retrospective assignment of blame.[30]

Because a hospital's board of trustees is inescapably part of the complex system of hospital care and because it can play a central role in fostering a culture of safety rather than a culture of blame, its members can be said to have moral responsibility—in the prospective sense—for health care quality within the institution.[31]

Thus, to say that error and, further, safety are "emergent properties of a system" and to recognize the inevitable role that humans play in designing and reacting to the system, is to place responsibility squarely on the shoulders of the collective to improve aspects of the system that are poorly designed, dysfunctional, or counterproductive. The legitimate expectation of patients that they will be helped and not harmed in this system is the moral basis of this responsibility.[32]

Given that trustees have strong external as well as internal motivations for advancing quality and patient safety in their institutions, how exactly should they go about it? A brief look at the theory of continuous quality improvement (CQI) provides some insight.

In the late 1980s, the theory of CQI, also known as "total quality management," began to replace the theory of quality assurance (QA) in health care. As Berwick observed it in his influential *New England Journal of Medicine* article "Continuous Improvement as an Ideal in Health Care,"[33] the theory of quality assurance assumes that quality fails when people do the right things wrong. As a result, QA depends on established standards as a gauge for performance evaluation, surveillance, and deterrence through penalties for noncompliance. CQI, by contrast, assumes that quality fails because people do the wrong things right. The aim of CQI is to identify the ways in which poor system design facilitates or fails to prevent potentially harmful errors.

The key to the implementation of CQI in health care institutions is attention to the processes of care that contribute to outcomes.[34] These include the flow of patients, for example, in admission, discharge, testing; the flow of information in appointments, referrals, test ordering, and informed consent; the flow of material, as in pharmacy and blood product dispensing and chart availability; and the interpersonal style of providers—their ability to listen, to communicate effectively, and to work in a team. CQI makes use of flowcharts, feedback diagrams, and other tools of industrial management to understand, predict, and improve processes. CQI is a "total" quality approach in that it integrates quality-related efforts horizontally across interdepartmental processes and vertically, across hierarchical levels.

This vertical integration both assumes and reinforces the central role that boards play in improving the quality of the institution's work. It also underscores that the achievement of quality is not simply a function of individual, but, rather, of collective responsibility. Like its industrial complement, "organizational learning," CQI is based on systems thinking. As management guru Peter Senge says, "In mastering systems thinking, we give up the assumption that there must be an individual, or individual agent responsible. The feedback perspective suggests that everyone shares responsibility for problems generated by a system. That doesn't necessarily imply that everyone involved can exert equal leverage in changing the system. But it does imply that the search for scapegoats . . . is a blind alley."[35] The IOM report recommendations emphasize the techniques of CQI as a basis for engendering a culture of safety in health care.

Boards can take a number of steps to become more involved in supporting and overseeing quality initiatives in their institution. Drawing on observation by Bryan Weiner and Jeffrey Alexander, the board can draft a "quality mission statement"[36] and communicate that message to staff. It can institute and financially sustain CQI training at all levels of the organization; it can form a "quality council" that studies and improves processes in light of institutionally determined goals; it can reinforce quality initiatives with a reward structure for executives.[37]

Integrating patient safety into these initiatives will require the institution to create opportunity and incentives for health care personnel candidly to discuss and learn from near misses as well as harmful error. This will involve partnership between malpractice carriers for the institution and risk managers, all of whom must support disclosure of information in the quality improvement process. Likewise, boards should assist clinicians and others in the caregiving process through training and support to overcome the psychological and emotional barriers to disclosure of error. The board should develop an explicit policy supporting disclosure of information to harmed patients and their families and should involve patients and families in safety committees.

Boards must recognize that quality improvement in this area cannot be achieved at the expense of the harmed patient's right to know. Boards must also be involved in the identification of specific safety indicators that will allow it to assess institutional performance over time. The board's role, in other words, must not simply be reactive to information supplied by the chief executive officer. Rather, boards must be proactive in taking and strategically directing action toward the improvement of patient safety.[38]

The role of hospital boards in patient safety is inescapable from both an ethical and a legal point of view. As the IOM recommendations are translated into regulatory requirements, this role will increase. The theory of continuous quality improvement shows great promise in its approach to institutional quality management. One of its most important precepts is that quality depends upon meeting the needs of patients. As boards take a more active role in patient safety within their institutions, they must recognize this as the guiding value of health care. A health care institution's mission is thus broader than its current legal and regulatory accountabilities. The best institutions have it as their guiding purpose and chief responsibility—at all levels—to keep faith with the ancient maxim "to help or at least to do no harm."

NOTES

1. Linda T. Kohn, Janet M. Corrigan, Molla S. Donaldson, eds., for the Institute of Medicine, Committee on Quality of Health Care in America, *To Err Is Human: Building a Safer Health System* (Washington, D.C.: National Academy Press, 1999). Available at www.quic .gov/Report/errors6.pdf.

2. Kohn et al., *To Err Is Human*, 1.

3. Kohn et al., *To Err Is Human*, 135.

4. Kohn et al., *To Err Is Human*, 135.

5. James E. Orlikoff and Mary K. Totten, *The Board's Role in Quality Care* (Chicago: American Hospital Publishing Inc., 1991).

6. Charles E. Rosenberg, *The Care of Strangers: The Rise of America's Hospital System* (New York: Basic Books, 1987).

7. Rosenberg, *Care of Strangers*, 271.

8. J. G. Bowman, "Hospital Standardization Series: General Hospitals of 100 or More Beds, Report for 1919," *Bulletin of the American College of Surgeons* 4 (1920): 3–36.

9. Virginia A. Sharpe and Alan I. Faden, *Medical Harm: Historical, Conceptual, and Ethical Dimensions of Iatrogenic Illness* (New York: Cambridge University Press, 1998). For a discussion of the elements of health care quality, see A. Donabedian, *Explorations in Quality Assessment and Monitoring*, 3 vols. (Ann Arbor, Mich.: Health Administration Press, 1980–85).

10. This view is expressed often in the literature of hospital administration. E.g., in 1947, G. G. Ward asserted that "the product of the hospital is health, and . . . we know that it is the character of the medical staff that determines the product of the hospital." In 1993, a physician-ethicist averred that "in the end, the patient's greatest guarantee of quality of care is the physician's character." See George G. Ward, "Audits Measure Our Results," *Modern Hospital* 69 (1947): 86; and Peter E. Dans, "Clinical Peer Review: Burnishing a Tarnished Icon," *Annals of Internal Medicine* 118, no. 7 (1993): 566–68.

11. *Darling v. Charleston Community Memorial Hospital* (1965) 33 Ill. 2d 326 [211 N.E. 2d 253, 14 A.L.R. 3d 860]. This case builds on the precedent set in *Bing v. Thunig* 2 N.Y.2d 656; 143 N.E.2d 3; 1957 N.Y. 163 N.Y.S.2d 3 1957, which established that the doctrine of charitable immunity from liability—first declared in *McDonald v. Massachusetts General Hospital* 120 Mass. 432 (1876)—is no longer applicable to hospitals. As the New York Court of Appeals observed, "there is general agreement among text writers and other commentators that the rule of immunity should be abandoned and the doctrine of *respondeat superior* reaffirmed to render the hospital liable for the torts of its employees" (at p. 21).

12. *Darling v. Charleston Community Memorial Hospital*, 332.

13. *Johnson v. Misericordia Community Hospital* 99 Wis. 2d 708; 301 N.W. 2d 156 1981 Wisc, 725.

14. Joseph O'Connor and Ian McDermott, *The Art of Systems Thinking: Essential Skills for Creativity and Problem Solving* (London: Thorsons, 1977).

15. G. Steven Wilkerson, "Hospital Trusteeship and Philanthropy in America," paper delivered at the Hastings Center / New York Academy of Medicine, Not-For-Profit Hospital Trustees Project Meeting IV, October 29–30, 1998.

16. Joint Commission on Accreditation of Healthcare Organizations, "The Agenda for Change," *Agenda Change Update* 1 (1987): 1–3.

17. Kohn et al., *To Err Is Human*, 59.

18. Laurie Larson, "Ending the Culture of Blame," *Trustee*, February 2000, 7; hyperlink at www.trusteemag.com.

19. Hippocrates, "Epidemics I," in *Hippocrates*, trans. W. H. S. Jones, Loeb Classical Library (Cambridge, Mass.: Harvard University Press, 1923–88), 165.

20. Virginia A. Sharpe, "'No Tribunal Other than His Own Conscience': Historical Reflections on Error and Responsibility in Medicine," *Proceedings of the National Patient Safety Foundation Conference on Enhancing Patient Safety and Reducing Errors in Health Care* (Chicago: National Patient Safety Foundation, 1999); Virginia A. Sharpe, "Behind Closed Doors: Accountability and Responsibility in Patient Care," *Journal of Medicine and Philosophy* 25, no. 1 (2000): 28–47. See also K. Darr, B. B. Longest Jr., and J. S. Rakich, "The Ethical Imperative in Health Services Governance and Management," *Hospital and Health Service Administration* 31, no. 2 (1986): 53–66. Of course, hospital trustees are presently understood to have fiduciary duties; however, these are traditionally understood to be duties of loyalty to the purpose for which the organization was created, not duties to patients per se.

21. M. S. Bogner, ed., *Human Error in Medicine* (Hillsdale, N.J.: Erlbaum, 1994). Also see R. I. Cook, D. D. Woods, and C. Miller, *A Tale of Two Stories: Contrasting Views of Patient Safety* (Chicago: National Patient Safety Foundation, 1998); available at www.npsf.org/exec /report.html. And see Lucian L. Leape, "Error in Medicine," *Journal of the American Medical Association* 272 (1994): 1851–57. Finally, see David W. Bates, D. J. Cullen, N. Laird, et al., "Incidence of Adverse Drug Events and Potential Adverse Drug Events: Implications for Prevention," *Journal of the American Medical Association* 274 (1995): 29–34.

22. L. Curtin and R. L. Simpson, "Making the Worst of a Bad Situation," *Health Management Technology*, July 2000, 42.

23. O'Connor and McDermott, *Art of Systems Thinking*, 6.

24. L. L. Leape, D. W. Bates, D. J. Cullen, et al., for the ADE Prevention Study Group, "Systems Analysis of Adverse Drug Events," *Journal of the American Medical Association* 274 (1995): 35–43.

25. D. M. Berwick, "Continuous Improvement as an Ideal in Health Care," *New England Journal of Medicine* 320 (1989): 53–56.

26. Marshall Kapp, "Medical Error Versus Malpractice," *DePaul Journal of Health Care Law* 1 (1997): 751–69.

27. Kohn et al., *To Err Is Human*, 4.

28. R. J. Croteau and E. S. Loeb, "Sentinel Events and Root-Cause Analysis: A Workshop by the Joint Commission," in *Proceedings of the National Patient Safety Foundation Conference on Enhancing Patient Safety and Reducing Errors in Health Care* (Chicago: National Patient Safety Foundation, 1999).

29. J. M Juran and F. M. Gryna, eds., *Juran's Quality Control Handbook*, 4th ed. (New York: McGraw-Hill, 1988); W. E. Deming, *Out of the Crisis* (Cambridge, Mass.: MIT Center for Applied Engineering Studies, 1986); D. Berwick, "Taking Action to Improve Safety: How to Increase the Odds of Success," in *Proceedings of the National Patient Safety Foundation Conference on Enhancing Patient Safety and Reducing Errors in Health Care* (Chicago: National Patient Safety Foundation, 1999).

30. Virginia A. Sharpe, "Taking Responsibility for Medical Mistakes," in *Margin of Error: The Ethics of Mistakes in the Practice of Medicine*, ed. S. Rubin and L. Zoloth-Dorfman (Frederick, Md.: University Publishing Group, 2000).

31. In this chapter, I assume that patient safety is a necessary subset of quality of care. Quality is the ability of an institution to serve patients' health interests. Safety is service to those interests without accidental injury; see Kohn et al., *To Err Is Human*, 3.

32. Virginia A. Sharpe, "Why 'Do No Harm'"? *Theoretical Medicine* 18 (1997): 197–216.

33. Berwick, "Continuous Improvement as an Ideal in Health Care."

34. G. Laffel and D. Blumenthal, "The Case for Using Industrial Quality Management Science in Health Care Organizations," *Journal of the American Medical Association* 83 (1989): 1031–37.

35. Peter Senge, *The Fifth Discipline: The Art and Practice of the Learning Organization* (New York: Currency Doubleday, 1994), 78.

36. Bryan Weiner and Jeffrey Alexander, "Hospital Governance and Quality of Care: A Critical Review of Transitional Roles," *Medical Care Review* 50, no. 4 (1993): 375–410.

37. David Classen, "Patient Safety, Thy Name Is Quality," *Trustee*, October 2000; www .trusteemag.com/asp/ArticleDisplay.asp?PubID = 3&ArticleID = 12972.

38. Shari Mycek, "Patient Safety: It Starts with the Board; When It Comes to the Fundamentals, Patient Safety Tops the List," *Trustee*, May 2001; www.trusteemag.com/asp/inside .asp?Type = articledisplay&ArticleID = 14305.

CONTRIBUTORS

Jeffrey A. Alexander is the Richard Carl Jelinek Professor of Health Management and Policy in the School of Public Health, University of Michigan.

Charles J. Dougherty is president of Duquesne University, Pittsburgh.

Joseph J. Fins is chief of the division of medical ethics, and professor of medicine and public health at Weill Medical College of Cornell University.

Alan R. Fleischman is senior vice president of the New York Academy of Medicine.

Bradford H. Gray is director of the Division of Health and Science Policy at the New York Academy of Medicine.

Bruce Jennings is senior research scholar at The Hastings Center and teaches at the Yale University School of Public Health.

Anthony R. Kovner is professor of health policy and management at the Wagner School of New York University.

Frances S. Margolin is director of community health programs and is responsible for the Community Care Network Demonstration Program at the Health Research and Education Trust / American Hospital Association, Chicago.

William F. May is Cary M. Maguire Professor of Ethics Emeritus at Southern Methodist University, Dallas, and fellow of the Institute of Practical Ethics and Public Life, University of Virginia, Charlottesville.

Mary A. Pittman is the president of the Health Research and Educational Trust / American Hospital Association, Chicago.

Elizabeth Robilotti is a doctoral student in the history and ethics of public health and medicine at Columbia University, New York.

David Rosner is the director of the Center for the History and Ethics of Public Health and professor of history and public health, Mailman School of Public Health, Department of Sociomedical Sciences, Columbia University, New York.

J. David Seay is the executive director of the National Alliance for the Mentally Ill of New York State and was formerly counsel for the United Hospital Fund of New York.

Virginia A. Sharpe is a visiting scholar at the Georgetown University Center for Clinical Bioethics. She was formerly deputy director of The Hastings Center.

David H. Smith is Nelson Poynter Senior Scholar and emeritus professor of religious studies at Indiana University, Bloomington.

Linda Weiss is a senior research associate in the Office of Special Populations at the New York Academy of Medicine.

Romana Hasnain-Wynia is the director, Research and Evaluation with the Health Research and Educational Trust / American Hospital Association, Chicago.

INDEX

Pages numbers followed by "f" denote figures; page numbers followed by "t" denote tables